Me 1 Arthritis 0

Me 1 Arthritis 0

◆

A Young Man's Real Life Journey to Beating the Disease

Brandon Wilkinson

iUniverse, Inc.
New York Bloomington Shanghai

Me 1 Arthritis 0
A Young Man's Real Life Journey to Beating the Disease

iUniverse books may be ordered through booksellers or by contacting:

iUniverse
1663 Liberty Drive
Bloomington, IN 47403
www.iuniverse.com
1-800-Authors (1-800-288-4677)

ISBN: 978-0-595-48824-7 (pbk)
ISBN: 978-0-595-48905-3 (cloth)
ISBN: 978-0-595-60859-1 (ebk)

Printed in the United States of America

Contents

Acknowledgments vii

Introduction ix

A Downward Spiral

Diagnosis 3

The Car Ride from Hell 6

Why Me? 9

Don't Give Me Your Pity! 21

Emotional Rollercoaster 25

Relationships 28

Private Health Care 33

Recuperation 38

Hope 43

South of the Border 44

Drink, Drugs and Tobacco 66

Chronic Pain—In the Ass 76

Lightweight 78

Sandy the Faith Healer 82

Live or Die 88

Talk to Me 104

Visit Back Home 105

The Upward Spiral Revival

The Land of Opportunity 111

A New Beginning? 123

I Love Your Accent 127

The Wonder Drug 136

Back on the Pies 143

Me, Myself and I 147

Haven't I Seen You Somewhere Before? 149

The Grand Slam 159

An Early Confession 161

It's a Wonderful Life 164

Moving In 165

Golfer Again 167

Finally on Track 178

Present Day 180

Acknowledgments

Firstly, with regard to the book title, the "me" part *is* actually referring to me. I was diagnosed with arthritis in my very early twenties. It had an alarming effect on my mind and emotions in general, and was definitely the most challenging segment of my life so far.

Me 1 Arthritis 0 is a real life account, which depicts my journey from diagnosis until present day. Life is a complicated struggle and I believe my inner feelings are shown in detail throughout this work; something that has basically been bottled up for many years.

The writing of this story was also a journey, which caused a multitude of emotions to continuously flood back to my mind. I cried, laughed, felt sad, as well as satisfied as I worked my way through the pages. The story is often dark, but filled with amusing anecdotes and tales that can be enjoyed by all.

Those out there who have experienced chronic pain and the adverse affects it can have on the mind will no doubt be intrigued. The emotional turmoil it can cause is experienced by most, so don't feel isolated, wondering what is happening to you—it is as ordinary as the common cold.

Like my first book, my wife and family were the driving force behind this latest piece of work. My father asked me what my inspiration was behind *Memoirs of the Messed Up Minds*. When I replied that my illness and the emotional effects were the motivation, he asked if I'd thought about telling my own story as opposed to creating fictional ones; I hadn't, but it was all I needed to hear to begin the tale of my woes.

To my wife Teri; I love you loads and you're always behind me in these efforts that often remove much of our time together. Of course a huge thank you to my dad, John and my mum, Betty who have supported me throughout my life and were the ones who cared for me during the tough times and put up with my mood swings and emotional outbursts.

Cheers to my younger brother Alan. I know he felt my pain also, and was always there for me and still is. When I was at my sickest it was as though he became the big brother, looking out for me and acting as my protector during my times of frailness and vulnerability.

To my other family members and friends; without your support I honestly don't know if I would be here today to share this story.

One final thanks to Melina for her time and effort reviewing this work and providing crucial inputs.

Laughter, tears, sympathy and joy are just a few of the emotions you will endure reading this book. I hope you enjoy it as much as I did writing it.

Included below are two photographs. I am a great believer that a picture says a thousand words. I feel that these will give you a sound perspective as you progress through the story.

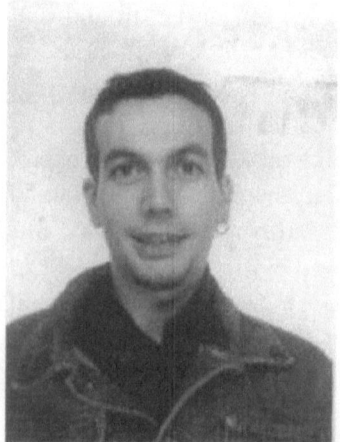

That Was Then
I was wilting away and down to a scary 106lbs. To say I was self-conscious would've been an understatement. The pain was so bad it eliminated any appetite. Even then I'd still try and force a smile for the camera.

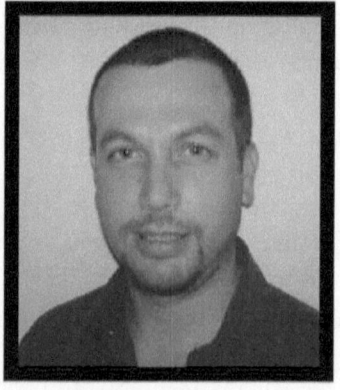

This Is Now
Pain is gone, weight is back to normal, and loving life again. It is so important to fight as long as it takes. I wouldn't be the mentally strong person I am today had I not endured this painful journey.

Introduction

This is not the typical run of the mill text you'd usually find in book stores across the country relating to arthritis. I am not a doctor providing commentary on advanced treatments or an infomercial host detailing other miraculous remedies. I am, however, an arthritis sufferer who was diagnosed with the condition in my early twenties, over ten years ago.

The story begins with my moment of diagnosis, before flashing back to my first indications of knee pain. It then continues on through my life journey until the present day, where I find myself essentially living a pain free existence.

Nowadays much of the focus—as it should be—is on the treatment of the physical side of the disease and the pain management aspect. Less attention seems to be dedicated to the mental and emotional struggles that go hand in hand. The emotional stress that the illness caused me was as tough to handle as the influx of chronic pain.

It was a time in my life when I was looking to settle down into a normal loving relationship, but found the mental baggage brought on by the disease made it virtually impossible for that to happen. Who would want to end up tied-down to a guy who could be potentially crippled by his late thirties? Much of the book chronicles these concerns.

There is a comedic element littered throughout the text that is at times sarcastic and edgy. I had to maintain humor in my life or I may have fallen completely into the depths of despair and unable to pull myself out again.

Enjoy.

A Downward Spiral

Diagnosis

To describe it as a bombshell would've been the understatement of my life. The numbness that filled my legs was immediate, and closely followed by a pounding in my chest never before experienced. It was like a magnified version of my heartbeat prior to entering the cold and nerve filled room of my final University exam. Back then the feeling was one of severe importance, knowing how life-changing the outcome of my performance would mean. It was the same this time, but in an existence altering way I'd never even considered during my entire twenty three years of being on this now cruel and twisted planet.

Doctor Marshall's lips were moving, but the numbness had spread to my mind, and I became a temporary deaf mute, understanding none of the obviously painful words coming from his mouth, and unable to reply even if I'd been able to comprehend.

Arthritis! What was the deal with that, surely there was a mistake. Wasn't that something reserved for old folks and retired football players who'd spent their prolonged careers on the injury report, renowned for taking a beating on the field when they were actually able to play?

I sat motionless, the room now spinning out of control, on par with my level of sanity. I was glad I was seated as he informed me how bad things really were. If not, I would've been crumpled on the floor like a pile of old clothes. That would've been as well to be the case, as my limbs were becoming useless, and further deterioration was likely to be high up on the future menu of life.

The diagnosis was bad enough, but the requirement for an almost immediate hip replacement was almost too much to take. I was a fighter though and always had been, but no amount of guts and determination could hold back the tears. They ran like a shakily written number eleven down my warm red cheeks, and I let out a huge sigh as my overwhelmed head sank wearily into my sweaty palms, fingers gripping on for dear life to my painfully moist and exhausted face. Doctor Marshall was silent, knowing I needed a moment to gather myself from the initial shock.

Doctor Marshall was a wonderful man who oozed confidence and success, yet the most down to earth and level headed physician I'd ever encountered. Our previous meeting had come as a surprise. I knew something was wrong with my knee and hip, but for some reason was referred to him by the Orthopedic Surgeon. I figured it was an injury I'd received from my martial arts training, and a quick twenty minute surgery to clean out some loose cartilage particles would have me back to the business of tearing up my weekly sparring partners. Finding nothing of that nature and sending me to a Rheumatologist for further tests was a slight surprise, but figured it was just the process of elimination that I was required to go through.

Like the whole Arthritis concept, I'd visualized this Rheumatologist by the name of Doctor Marshall to be a crusty looking older chap, no stranger to a bit of joint pain himself, but he was a complete contrast the first time we met, nattily dressed, fully functional, Gucci spectacles, and a hair style complimenting the ability of any high class salon.

"Mr. Wilkinson, what can I do you for?" he said in a cheerful tone that set me at ease immediately. This was *my* type of doctor, down to earth, bit of working class patter, and a warmness about him that let you know he was there for you and not just the substantial monetary element that went hand in hand with seeing a physician of his stature and reputation.

"My knee's swollen and I'm getting a bit of irritation in the old hip here," I said pointing rather awkwardly to my left hip socket.

"Jump up on the table here and let me take a look," he said pleasantly, like it was just another routine examination, and I'd be out of there in no time with a prescription for some pain killers and fatherly advice to "take it easy for a while."

He pushed my limbs around like a rag doll and I flinched abruptly, as he took it a little too far in my immediate opinion. I quickly thought, "I can usually do that" but the pain was incredible. I was known as the "rubber man" at my martial arts class, many of the male students seeming envious, probably in the thought that I could've actually performed fellatio on myself, much to their mistake. If that'd been the case, I'd have been an absentee on a regular basis from the weekly class!

"Wow, easy there tiger," I said to Dr. Marshall, twisting out of the gymnastic move he was pulling on me.

"Mmm," he said with a baffling tone.

"Mmm?" I replied, directing it as a question rather than a witty response.

"Stand up for a second and touch your toes."

I eagerly jumped off the solid surface of the "bed" and reached down with my finger tips towards the end of my black leather shoes. It was a struggle as I let out a groan, commonly heard from older men reaching to pick up money that spilled from their pockets. Holy crap, I'd always been able to do this with ease, and was only ever a centimeter or so from achieving the splits.

He looked thoughtful, as though he'd suddenly been asked to solve a complex calculus equation. He felt my right knee again, which felt warm to me and was swollen like a helium filled balloon. Reaching into the drawer of his oak looking desk, he pulled out a syringe and a tiny bottle of white liquid that he drew from with the needle and asked me to pull up my trouser leg.

"And this would be what?" I asked, extremely alarmed with the sudden action.

"You've got some serious inflammation in your knee joint, and this will help it go away."

I loved layman's terms. "This will help it go away" was all I needed to hear. That was what I was here for after all, to make the pain go away.

The syringe entered me almost unnoticed, as I casually looked out of the window at the hustle and bustle of life going around, unaware of my current situation—until the needle penetrated my knee joint. It burst through like the popping of a piece of bubble wrap, causing me to flinch and almost heel kick myself in my innocent left shin bone.

"Holy shit Doc, wasn't expecting that."

'I'm sorry, but that's why I don't tell, it is painful, but I need you relaxed, I need to be precise," he uttered, delivering the thick white liquid to my unsuspecting joint. That was even more painful, and felt like it was squeezing an obese gentleman into a dwarf's closet.

"Wow," was the only word I could state, trying to maintain every piece of manliness I'd ever inherited.

That was just the beginning, as he took a blood sample from the bulging vein from the opposite side of my right elbow.

"You're earning your money today Doc," I gasped, as the slender needle was removed from my pulsating arm.

"Just need to send off a sample for the lab, there's a chance it could be arthritis."

Arthritis, yeah right, I'm a young man.

Those words of doubt certainly came back to bite me.

The Car Ride from Hell

My legs were still weary from the initial shock, and the joint pain was more intense than ever before. Maybe the mental realization of the cause was the contributing factor. The human psyche was a powerful beast and there was no hiding from it now behind my previous barrier of denial. I hated hospital parking lots—there were never enough spaces. For the first time in my life I wished I was the holder of a disabled badge as I passed the many spaces adjacent to the entrance. An elderly gentleman in his late sixties beeped the alarm on his vehicle from one of the spots—why did he have a pass? He was dressed typically for his age, uncoordinated with his brown pants and non-matching blue shirt, belt line almost under his armpits like he'd jumped off the wardrobe to get into the wrinkled trousers. He was very upbeat, whistling as he briskly made his way to the automatic double doors of the entrance. He gave me a strange look as he passed, almost obnoxious in the way his brow furrowed at the sight of my struggle. I paused to return the stare, but his brow ironed out and was replaced by a fake smile and acknowledgment of my pain as his eyebrows raised and he quickly disappeared into the building never to be seen again. I couldn't see my car but knew the rough direction, lost in the ant like crowd in the distance.

Like a typical Scottish day, the wind howled as I shakily headed on my way; it was almost emphasizing the life long journey that was ahead of me, not just now, but for many years to come. Each step seemed like ten yards as I headed wearily in the direction I prayed was correct. My limp was almost magnified now and I felt as though I was dragging my hip torn leg more than ever. A car horn sounded as I was halfway across one of the car park rows, and I felt the hairs on my neck stand on end like a troop of elite soldiers. I turned to my left to see an impatient looking overweight woman—no doubt undeservedly making her way to the disabled section—giving me a look that would've turned the dead in their graves. She had a child wailing like a banshee in the back seat, undoubtedly contributing to her impatience.

Go screw yourself you fat cow, can't you see I'm struggling here.
I greeted her delightful introduction with a swift middle finger salute.
I might be frail and in pain, but I can still take you in a scrap you plump old bag.

She continued on her way, but I prayed she would stop and display her obvious annoyance to me, but much to my dissatisfaction she proceeded down the road. I was ready for her as well, but like the previous part of my day, nothing transpired like I'd hoped it would. With a bit of luck the screaming child would continue on for the remainder of the afternoon and give her the type of feeling I was currently going through!

I finally arrived at the car, sweating profusely and aching all over. It was only about three hundred yards from the hospital entrance, but in arthritis years it was as though I'd matched Sir Edmund Hillary and conquered Everest. One of Hillary's famous quotes flashed in my mind *"It is not the mountain we conquer but ourselves."* Arthritis was now my mountain, but I had to fight through my inner trauma. It would be an uphill battle, but I was prepared to pull on the gloves, throw in the mouth guard, and charge in swinging.

Those thoughts brought a slight hint of a smile to my scrawny looking face—although the fact I was now seated in a warm vehicle with the stress removed from my joints was probably a contributing factor also.

I attempted to remain positive as I lazily drove towards home, spacing out into a complete haze as I reflected on my former life.

I used to be a fine physical specimen all throughout my life. I excelled in any sport that involved a ball, and was the envy of many in the way I could successfully interchange between activities, and was labeled with various nicknames over the years relating to my speed and agility.

Forest Gump was one I was tagged with when I played field hockey. I would knock the ball beyond the opposition defenders and sprint past them like a greyhound; the chants of "run Forest, run" from my friends on the sidelines only motivating me to retrieve the ball, which I never failed to do.

Even as a naïve twelve year old I was known as Koala, in light of my ability to quickly climb any tree in the forest adjacent to my parent's house. I was scared of nothing as I reached heights of fifty feet, interchanging branches like Tarzan; I was unaware of the potential danger should one of the limbs suddenly break. Looking back on this it was verging on idiotic, but I was happy, free as a bird, and just plain loving life. Not anymore!

I quickly awakened from my trance. I must've driven about a mile and hadn't remembered any of the journey so far; I was on complete auto-pilot. I drove leisurely, there was no point in rushing like a madman, wasn't like I had a full night of strenuous activities on the agenda. My lackluster pace seemed to be annoying the hell out of the others on the road, as a gradually increasing line was forming behind me—and I was doing the speed limit! The guy behind me was particularly frustrated. Visible in my rear view mirror, he appeared to be gradually boiling, his face initially your typical milk bottle white Scottish appearance, but within a matter of minutes he appeared as though someone had been using his head as target practice in a plum throwing contest. He would swerve out to overtake, only to jerk back in behind me to avoid oncoming traffic. He was a complete nutcase, with features to match—shaved, bald fat head, thick eyebrows like a couple of hairy caterpillars, and apparently no evidence of a neck. Maybe he was a football hooligan, associated with one of the local Glasgow clubs. I didn't care though. What was he going to do, pull me over and kick the crap out of me? Maybe so, but I was used to pain; and perhaps he'd be doing me a favor if he put me out of my misery. He was riding my bumper frighteningly close. If it wasn't for his windshield I was convinced he could've punched me on the back of the head right there and then. Finally he saw his opportunity and screeched past me at a rapid rate of knots, pulling in tightly in front of me not a moment too soon, closely avoiding an oncoming black Ford. The occupant of the vehicle, an elderly looking grey haired woman had a look of horror on her face as she whizzed past. If she didn't smell of urine already, she certainly did now. Fat head continued on his way after flicking me off, but that was the least of my worries.

Traffic was heavy and I seemed to catch every red light possible—nothing was going my way today. The sun began to appear from behind a dark, rain threatening cloud, perhaps a sign of brighter things to come in my life, but I wasn't seeing it. As I sat at each light, I surveyed the people on the streets going about their daily lives. They all seemed unusually happy, as mothers pushed their young children around gleefully in their strollers, kids played and had a perky spring in their steps, and joggers jaunted past merrily to the beat entering their heads from their iPod running companions. That used to be me. Fit as a fiddle, spring in *my* step, joyfully going about my daily business, and looking forward to the following day.

Eventually I arrived home at my parents place, mentally exhausted and looking forward to the hike up the stairs to their third floor apartment! They were going to be stunned by the news. They loved me more than life itself, and I knew they'd be there for me, but I always thought I'd be the one who would end up taking care of them, not the other way around. I sobbed my heart out as I prepared for the painful and exhausting slog to their front door.

Why Me?

Had I been a bad person who deserved this punishment? I racked my brains to find a reason, but I'd always been a law abiding citizen. Don't get me wrong, as a young teenager I'd had my share of questionable behavior, but who hadn't! Once I'd been put in detention at high school when I was thirteen, after being caught by the headmaster giving my English teacher a masturbation hand gesture behind his back. He *was* a wanker though, and I was just a stupid kid following the crowd of others who'd done the same before me, but I just happened to be the one who was caught in the act.

There was one other time around a similar age that my buddies and I played a game of "light a shite" in one of the elderly housing communities near my home. I'd wrapped a large piece of dog shit in toilet paper, set it on fire on a cold front doorstep and knocked on the door heavily before running around the corner. Our hilarity hit new heights as the frail old man opened the door, was consumed with panic, and began stamping on it like an over zealous Irish dancer. He wasn't even wearing shoes either!

That was about the extent of my misbehavior. I was a good student, breezing through high school and similarly with University. It made my skin crawl to know that there were many rapists and pedophiles running around this country without even a sign of an ailment other than their twisted sick minds. Where was the justice? It was at this point that my belief in a higher power was abandoned completely, and I sided with the theory of evolution from that day forward.

I tried to sleep at nights, I really did, but my mind was racing. Would I really be a cripple in about ten years? Looking down at my skinny legs as I lay on the burgundy feathered comforter, I concluded that it was a distinct possibility. My previous muscle bound, martial arts style legs had already been replaced by those resembling a chicken, and not even a tough one at that! I was becoming frail, unable to fully extend my right leg, and the muscle around the knee-cap steadily withering away into oblivion.

I would hear every creak and noise from outside as I lay in my lonely bedroom half hoping it was from a psychopathic burglar invading my residence, stabbing me in the heart as I discovered his presence. At least that would've given me an escape route without having to take my own life. They would've mourned me proudly, knowing I'd likely put up an almighty fight considering my condition.

I was losing my mind.

No you're not!

All my irrational fears and concerns were pouring out. Fortunately the voice of the "old" me was still inside my head, struggling to keep me on the straight and narrow, dragging me away from the edge of the emotionally damaging cliff-top.

Maybe I *should* just end my life, save myself the future pain and suffering—might be doing everyone a favor, particularly my family. At least I'd be saving them the mental anguish of watching my deterioration, wilting away to a state of nothingness.

They love you, get a hold of yourself. There have been a lot of good times, and there will be many again. Stop being such a selfish little coward.

There was such a feeling of déjà vu as I lay in bed at night. The empty, dull and lifeless white ceiling was always the same, and about as colorful as my present existence. I'd cast my mind back to good times from the past; triumphant soccer games, winning golf tournaments and kicking and punching my way to a success in local martial arts competitions; all fun times, but requiring levels of physical ability that were now beyond me. I did have the memories of success, which was probably more than many ever would. I'd smile as I visualized the game ending goal, winning putts, not to mention a firm right sidekick to an unsuspecting opponent's mid-section.

I was careful not to move around on the mattress though as I replayed these visions in my head, every twitch resulting in shooting pain, a reminder of the uphill struggle ahead of me.

I really had to start eating more, I was definitely losing weight, but like nicotine, pain was one sure way of repressing an appetite, and the thought of enduring the short walk to the kitchen was about as appealing as a hearty meal. It was a similar feeling to that of being heartbroken; a gut wrenching phenomenon that I'd experienced not too long before now. That sick feeling in my stomach had returned, and brought those hurtful emotions racing back into the forefront of my mind.

I was a fit and healthy eighteen year old, brimming with confidence now that I was a University student, and had my whole life ahead of me to accomplish whatever I set my mind to; or so I thought at the time. She was in my Computing Science class, a daily vision that kept me motivated with a subject matter I really didn't care for. I so looked forward to seeing her smooth sallow skin, long flowing brown curls and sweet embarrassed looking smirk as she entered the lecture room a few minutes late. Her timekeeping skills left a lot to be desired, as she was usually the last person to enter the lecture theatre; much to my delight, as I got to study her perfect form and drift off into a temporary fantasy for a few minutes. It was comical in the way she almost tip-toed into class, aware of her lateness, even cartoon like, much like a mischievous Tom creeping up on an unsuspecting Jerry. Why our lecturer Dr. Steinberg wasn't as equally fascinated was beyond me; it was adorable. I automatically assumed he wasn't attracted to women.

He ran a tight ship, punctuality being of prime importance, and hated his dull ramblings being interrupted by latecomers, whether they were females of extreme beauty, or one of the fat lads from the back of the lecture hall who'd stopped off for an extra pie on the way to class. At least he was consistent I suppose.

Steinberg reminded me of Chewbacca, maybe the hairiest man on the face of the planet. He could have sunbathed on the beach and you'd have sworn he was still fully clothed. I was sure he had a face in there somewhere, but his beard was obviously a work in progress that had been going on for a couple of years. This was a typical look for many of the lecturers, together with a fashion sense that was stuck in a time warp. I was sure it was stylish back in the seventies, but certainly not in the nineties. He was a genius though, an eccentric one at that, and I doubt he really gave a crap what people thought of him anyway, which was actually an admirable quality.

Olga was her name. I found this out from a girl by the name of Gillian whom I used to work with in my Statistics class. She often sat beside Olga in the Computing lecture and had got to know her pretty well. I felt as though I was still in my early teenage years as I told Gillian I thought her new friend "was really cute" and to "put in a good word for me." I might have been confident, but the idea of rejection was a terrifying one, and this seemed like a safer approach.

I saw them both looking back at me one day in the Computing classroom; Gillian had obviously passed on my regards. My heart pumped as I quickly looked away, petrified that her assessment of me wouldn't meet her standards, which I assumed from her overall beauty would be fairly high on the probability scale. The hour long class felt like days as I contemplated what her verdict had been, feeling like the accused anxiously awaiting the return of the jury members.

Gillian was waiting for me outside the class after Steinberg's rants on the importance of Pascal programming to society finally ceased. Fortunately there was no sign of Olga, either not wanting to be there as Gillian informed me of the disappointment, or not wanting the embarrassment of being there for the "not proven" verdict.

I was like the Cheshire cat, smiling from ear to ear as Gillian delivered the news. It was a total result. She thought *I* was cute, and that I should go out with them on Thursday night, as they were heading into town for a drink. I didn't have to be asked twice, stating I'd be there. There was a small group heading out, and I invited my buddies Paul and Graham for added support, and also in case things didn't go according to plan. It was only two days away, but couldn't come quickly enough.

I washed and showered like a madman, finding crevasses and areas of skin never before encountered by my soap and sponge. I'd even substituted the typical "bar" of soap with some form of scented body wash gel—an unused Christmas present—that was gathering dust and cobwebs in the corner of the tiled wall, which itself hadn't seen a scrub with a cloth and bathroom cleaner in quite some time.

Be prepared was the motto for the night. There wasn't much chance of getting laid, in fact the bookmakers would probably have touted odds of about 1%, but that made all the difference.

So there's still a chance!

I toweled off and slipped on my best pair of clean Calvin Klein underwear. It's what my Mother would've wanted, albeit for a different motive—citing "in case you get into an accident" rather than the prospect of a fit young woman tearing them off with her teeth. That itself could potentially lead to an accident though, involving my ability of self-control, which might almost be as devastating from an embarrassment standpoint as being ploughed down by an oncoming motor vehicle!

I met up with Paul and Graham at Darcy's bar in Princess Square. People eye-balled us in detail as we entered the premises, me in the middle and my new University buddies either side. It was quite a site. I stood a *towering* five feet six inches, Paul was around six feet five, and Graham an equally respectable six two. Maybe the patrons thought I was someone important, with two bodyguards by my side—they couldn't have been more wrong. To make matters worse, neon lights filled the room, and I was clad in dark blue jeans and a bright orange silk shirt, and both the boys were all in black, from jeans, t-shirts, down to the almost matching leather jackets. I know they hadn't coordinated before coming out for the night, but it felt like they were involved in an elaborate practical joke to highlight my presence to Olga. That would've been fine, but we weren't meeting them at Darcy's. We were just stopping there for a couple of shots of Dutch courage before heading upstairs in this nighttime Plaza, to the "October Café."

Princess Square was a posh indoor shopping and restaurant area by day. At night it was a trendy hangout place, shops closed for the evening and the restaurants turning into cool night spots to enjoy a beverage. Food was still available, but grossly outweighed by the volume of beer and liquor that was flowing. It *was* Thursday after all—student night, which involved up and coming DJ's spinning tunes, but more importantly half-priced drinks on beer, or order a shot and receive a double measure. These were the two offers which caused me no end of amusement. Did the bar management really see a huge difference between "half price" and "two for one"!

After the couple of nerve conquering cold ones, we took the elevator to the top floor, the location of the October Café. The place was a beautiful one, with marble looking floors and shiny gold colored banisters lining all staircases. The place was bustling as we looked out over the setting from the glass elevator. The ride up was a speedy one, and caused the four beers to go straight to my head, creating a nice "buzz", giving me the feeling that everything was wonderful.

Rarely in Scotland does a couple of drinks actually imply that, although in this case they'd only cost me the price of a couple, so my conscience was clear. Billy Connolly summed Scottish drinking culture up best when he exclaimed "my wife thought a pint was this size" (simulating an object three times the size of a bucket). Every time he said to her he was "going for a pint," he would come home to her blind drunk.

We entered the October Café, my confidence from the beer buzz was swiftly replaced by extreme nerves and a sick feeling in my stomach as I caught a glimpse of my friend Gillian's unmistakable reddish orange hair as the strobe light from the almost disco setting lit her up like a firework. This meant that Olga was probably here also. We had never really spoken, so I was almost trembling, begging my inner self not to blurt out something of extreme stupidity as my first line. First impressions counted for a lot and a previous female friend had informed me that women decide within the first five minutes or so if they would be likely to sleep with a guy—that evening or anytime in the near future.

As we approached the gang I could see Olga there, back to us, but her long flowing brown locks of hair were unlike any other. My heart was pounding, but I had to appear confident.

"How you doing ladies?"

"Hey Brandon, late as usual I see," said Gillian, giving Olga a glance.

"Fashionably," I retorted.

"This is Olga," said Gillian.

Yeah, nice one Gillian! Don't bother to go around the others first; just go straight to the object of my desires.

"Hi there Olga, I've heard a lot about you," I said with a smile.

"Really!" she said, turning towards Gillian.

I was glad to take the heat off myself for a few seconds to gather my thoughts.

"Don't worry, it was all good," said Gillian rather quickly.

"Olga, it was; I was rather impressed actually," I interjected with a smirk.

"By the way, this is Sharon, Cecilia and Martin," said Gillian, eager to change the conversation, but I could tell Olga was wondering about previous chats that had occurred between Gillian and myself.

"Nice to meet you all. No offense Martin, I wasn't including you in the 'how you doing ladies' greeting."

"None taken," said Martin with a snigger.

"This is Graham and Paul," I said.

Everyone settled in and we ordered a round of drinks.

Sharon and Cecilia were really bubbly characters and I could tell they'd be a lot of fun. Sharon was about five seven, a healthy looking figure on her with shoulder length curly brown hair and full lips. Cecilia made me look like a giant; five feet tall on her tip-toes, face as cute as a button and complimented by her dazzling white teeth, and a chest so stacked it would've taken about an hour to kiss every inch of it.

It was a close contest between Olga and Cecilia for the "best breasts" award, but I gave Olga the title by a short nipple, mainly because my desire to see them in the flesh was verging on overpowering.

Martin was a quiet guy and I was beginning to feel a little sorry for him as he wasn't involved in any of the conversations that were going on. I suspected he didn't have many male friends due to the fact he went out alone with four females. They probably viewed him as one of them as he was very unthreatening in appearance and a little bit girly. He reminded me of the folks who frequented Star Trek conventions and the likes, with the middle parting in his hair, thick lens glasses like a couple of milk bottles and a tight pair of Wrangler jeans with the matching buttoned up shirt tucked firmly into the trousers.

"So Olga, how are things going with your classes?" I inquired, deciding to go with a safe conversation topic before eventually kicking it up a notch of two.

"Pretty good; I mean I wish I didn't have to study, but hopefully it'll work out in the long run."

'I'm sure you'll be fine. I've heard tales about how bright you are."

"Oh have you now; seems like you've heard quite a few things about me. Not sure I've been told quite as much about you."

"What would you like to know? I'm an open book."

"I'm not sure; I suck when I'm put on the spot."

It took every face muscle I had to prevent an outburst of laughter, and I fought to remove the mental image from my mind. I *was* putting her on the spot, and if she wanted to suck, I was ready, willing, and able!

"OK, let me ask you a question; do you like Chinese food?"

"Yes, Chinese and Indian are my favorites," she replied with a semi-baffled look.

"I know this really smart place called the China Blossom in the center of town. Maybe I could take you there for a nice dinner one night next week? I mean, no pressure, just some good food, intellectual conversation, and perhaps a couple of glasses of chilled white wine."

I was kicking it up a notch or two quicker than I had planned, but her body language had been extremely telling since I'd arrived; piercing glances and warm smiles, so I figured there was no time like the present.

"That sounds nice," she replied, as a faint trace of blushing appeared on her sallow skin.

Result! No problem to the Brandon boy.

"Cool, I'll talk to you about it on Monday and we can set something up," I replied, almost stammering my words in surprise. I wasn't quite expecting such a positive response straight off the bat, figuring I'd have to coax her into it a little bit first.

"Great, sounds like fun," she said, again showing off her perfectly formed smile.

"Right, let's finish up our drinks and head to a club," said Paul, taking charge of the proceedings.

I wasn't overly enthusiastic about clubbing, but this place wasn't too bad. I just felt that most nightclubs put a bit of a damper on conversation, due to the thunderous beats of the music that usually resulted in repeating your words, even to someone standing directly beside you.

This was a neat place though, even for those—such as me—who weren't overly enthusiastic about dancing. It wasn't so much that I didn't enjoy it, more my lack of coordination and stepping around as though I had two left feet; one of them wearing a clubbed shoe! Even when I got the balls together to get on the dance floor—a minimum requirement of six pints consumed—I would just flap around to the techno anthems like an epileptic on speed who was bursting for a piss!

They had a separate room off to the side called "The Chill Out Zone". It was well named, filled with comfy suede blue sofa's and chairs, romantic style lighting, and slow rhythmical R&B tunes played at a volume no louder than the local bar.

The girls were dancing though in the main bustling room while we guys slouched on a sofa and chair in the corner of the Chill Out Zone like four sacks of potatoes, shooting the breeze about the upcoming weekend soccer matches and swigging on some overpriced bottles of cold Budweiser.

The scenery was unbelievable. Every female was decked out in short skirts, tight tops and had obviously meticulously applied make-up and lipstick, and spruced up their hair for their evening parade. Olga was still firmly in my mind though and I eagerly awaited her return from the crazy dance floor.

The girls finally returned, seeming a little out of breath from the events with the over exuberant clubbers. Olga greeted me with a smile and I could see a faint sliver of sweat on her forehead. Her beautiful brown eyes had a glazed appearance, undoubtedly a result of the Vodka and Red Bull mixtures kicking in.

She perched herself on the arm of the sofa directly beside my end position, much to my excitement. She had other options of where to sit, but the fact she chose this particular location told me she was most definitely interested.

Gravity was a wonderful thing, as the soft arm of the sofa together with her body weight caused her to gradually slouch towards me, and was only halted as our outer thighs connected and she moved her hand onto my left leg to prevent slipping down even further—she didn't remove her hand. I could see the others sensing that something was brewing as they watched discreetly. The previous amber light had now changed to green and it was all systems go. I place my hand on top of hers and she responded by grasping it gently and we gave each other a lustful gaze.

The boys excused themselves, citing they were going to the bar for another round of drinks, and Gillian, Sharon, and Cecilia conveniently needed to go to the bathroom to "freshen up." I moved over slightly and Olga slid elegantly into my previous location. We were like two peas in a pod as we immediately locked ourselves in a passionate embrace. Our soft lips and tongues battled in a frantic game of tonsil hockey; the taste of Red Bull and sparkling sweat from her upper lip only adding to the eroticism.

Get in there my son!

That night would be etched in my mind forever, and our relationship gathered pace over the following months. It was my first *real* sexual relationship, and I was discovering things I thought were only true in Hollywood chick flicks. I loved her dearly and the feeling was mutual.

Olga's parents were from Greece, but had gone through a nasty divorce five years previously that resulted in her father moving back to Athens. Her mother had taken well to me, although from what Olga had told me, she'd been hoping she would've found a "nice Greek boy".

I wasn't quite as fortunate with her father—he detested me even though we'd never actually met. Race, color or creed was never something that entered my mind; I was an equal opportunity lover who just wanted to be with someone who I had a good mental connection with, and Olga was *the one* in my eyes. Her father's determination to keep it in the family—so to speak—was surprising in this day and age, and seemed to neglect any thoughts that his daughter might actually be happy with a "nice Scottish boy".

We finally got the opportunity to meet one evening. Her father was over on a two week vacation to catch-up with friends, and from Scotland, Olga was returning with him to Athens for two months over the summer—a prospect that was killing me inside. We never went a day without seeing each other, never mind two whole months! No doubt her father, Nikos, or "that sneaky wanker" as I often referred to him during conversations with friends—Olga not being present of course—would be working on her mind over there, trying to convince her I was bad news, or even attempt to hook her up with one of these "nice Greek boys" I kept hearing about.

I arrived nervously at Olga's house knowing her father was there. I was *so* conscious about making a good impression that my stomach was churning like crazy. Olga must've been on edge as well, as her face appeared at the living room window within seconds of the sound of my car door closing; only adding to my current anxiety levels.

I walked slowly up the gravel covered driveway towards the front door, frantically rehearsing my introduction and firm manly handshake in my head.

Nice to meet you sir; Olga's told me a lot of good things about you.

It was such lies, but maybe he'd change his tune after meeting me and realize I was a decent, educated character who loved his daughter dearly.

Olga greeted me at the door with a nervous, almost fake smile and a tighter hug than usual.

"I'm ready if you are," I said with a smirk and a roll of my eyes.

"He'll be nice," were her words, but with enough unconvincing execution that I knew she was just trying to put me at ease.

We entered the living room, her father sitting slouched on the armchair like Santa at his grotto, with a similar roly-poly type stomach—he was no stranger to a double helping of Mousaka! Her mother was on the adjacent leather couch, sitting forward on the very edge of the end cushion in anxious anticipation. From what I'd been told, mother and father couldn't stand being in each other's company, so no doubt my arrival was giving "Mum" additional mental anguish.

Nikos pulled his lazy ass out of the chair as I approached him.

"Nice to meet you sir; Olga's told me a lot of good things about you," I said, extending my hand for the obligatory shake.

Holy crap, his grip was like a vice, and it took me every ounce of self control not to react in pain. I couldn't tell if this was his normal force or whether it was an alpha dog attempt at letting me know not to mess with him.

"Nice to meet you; so what's Olga said about me then?"

That you're a control freak and generally a dick.

I wanted to say that, but was still in shock by his question, and the fact I was on the spot and the clock was ticking. My question had been a rhetorical one!

I stuttered and stammered.

"Well … well, she said you're a great father and just an overall good guy."

Yeah, quality line Brandon; sounded extremely genuine!

Before he could reply, "Mum" let out a huge sigh, obviously siding with my previous inner thoughts of him being a complete dick.

"Would everyone like a coffee?" interrupted Olga, doing her best to diffuse the ever growing awkwardness.

"Sounds great; I'll give you a hand," I said in super quick fashion, beating her mother to the punch—there was no way I was being left there alone with old misery guts.

As we left the living room and headed to the kitchen, her mother let out another huge sigh.

That was the one and only time I met her Dad, and left the house that evening feeling worse than when I'd arrived.

Olga arrived at my parents place looking even more beautiful than ever. I had mixed feelings about her visit as she was leaving for a summer in Greece the following morning. Our initial embrace had intensity to it like never before; we both knew our time apart was going to be difficult.

"I'm going to miss you," I said, gazing so deeply into her eyes that I could almost see her retina.

"Let's not talk about that right now," she replied; her eyes beginning to fill with tears.

My Mum and Dad liked Olga a lot, and had never hit *me* with the "we'd hoped you would have found a nice Scottish girl" line. They were just pleased I was happy.

After exchanging a few pleasantries with my folks, we escaped to the comfort of my room where the hugging, kissing, and gazing continued. I wanted to rip her clothes off right there and then and ravish her entire body, but with my parents being downstairs that wasn't a possibility.

We just lay there for hours, fully clothed on top of my royal blue quilt, snuggled up in each others arms. Conversation was at a bare minimum. We didn't want to discuss the ultimate departure, which was the only thing on our minds, so it was better to avoid the topic and savor the quiet loving encounter we were sharing. I never wanted this moment to end, but as I looked at my clock on the wall, its pointed hands appeared to be moving faster than usual, and closer to Olga's departure.

"I should really get going," she said nervously.

"I know," I replied, grasping her tightly in my arms, seemingly squeezing a sweet tear from each of her loving brown eyes.

I watched intently as they trickled down her smooth cheeks in perfect formation, and I wiped them away with my fingers as they were about to fall onto the quilt.

"Don't cry sweetheart, it'll be alright. I'll write to you everyday."

Four weeks passed, and I'd stuck to my words. I'd never been one for writing love letters before, but this girl was special. I was like a lost puppy without her, but kept myself as busy as possible in order to keep her absence out of my mind, but her pretty face always invaded my thoughts.

I was never much of a morning person, but that had all changed since she'd left, as I lay awake every morning by 7:00am, intently listening for the sound of the postman pushing open our mailbox. I'd been receiving a letter every other day, and I read every one of them at least three or four times. It warmed my heart to know she was still thinking about me and expressing her love, but in the back of my mind I knew her father would be tainting her thoughts as much as possible.

The familiar rattle of the mailbox had me at attention as usual and I scurried merrily down the stairs. My smile spread from ear to ear as I identified the Greek postmark on the crisp white envelope. I eagerly ripped it open and began to read. My joy quickly changed to panic and tears.

Dear Brandon,

This is perhaps the hardest thing I've ever had to write, and I apologize for not having the guts to tell you in person. I've thought long and hard about this and have had several sleepless nights, but feel I have to stand by my decision.

For the first couple of weeks we were apart I was missing you like crazy, but as time has passed by these feelings have been becoming weaker and weaker, so I believe we should break-up and start our lives again separately. I'm having fun over here and don't want to feel tied down right now by our relationship. The one thing our time apart has told me is that I am not ready for that level of commitment right now. I know this must be hurting you and I hate myself for doing this, but I don't want to go on living a lie. Hopefully in time you will understand and feel better about things.

Sorry,

Olga

I was frozen to the spot in disbelief; tears pouring from my eyes and I had a sick feeling in my stomach unlike anything I'd ever experienced before. My heart was pounding and I felt like I was going to pass out. I had lost her, my rock, my soul mate, and didn't believe that time would ever heal this sickness and pain.

My relationship with Olga had been several years before my arthritis diagnosis, and as she said, I did get better over time but I never thought I'd endure that gut wrenching sick feeling again—at least to the same degree, but I was now. The realization that I had contracted a degenerating disease with no known cure was crippling me inside as well as outside. How could time help me now? If anything, time was now my enemy. Why me?

Don't Give Me Your Pity!

My parents took the news pretty badly as I tentatively delivered it, attempting to appear as positive as possible, but they saw straight through it. My pain stricken face was a give away, and they'd always been able to read me like a book.

Their emotional overload spilled into tears, and I knew this was hurting them almost as much as it was me. They hugged me tighter than ever, almost python like. The feeling of their love was almost overbearing, and sent me over the edge as I joined their chorus of sobs. I didn't want to put this on them—they worried enough already when I would go out for a night on the town, consuming large quantities of alcohol. Glasgow was a well renowned city for late night drunken fights and stabbings.

"I wish it was me instead of you son," said my dad, fighting through his tears of love and concern.

This only added to my distress. They would climb the highest mountain and jump off any bridge if it meant making the life ahead of me a more comfortable and pleasant one. I was going to fight this and make them proud—they at least deserved that.

"I'm a fighter Dad. You can't keep a good man down," I said, with the hint of a chuckle edging its way through the tears.

My folks had always supported me to the hilt throughout my life. My dad had just turned fifty, but was an incredibly fit man for his years. He'd been a professional football player, career cut short by a horrendous knee injury. His hair was completely grey, and had been for some time—a genetic event that hit him from about thirty and would no doubt be inherited from my end. I was cool with that as I saw him as a fabulous role model. If I turned out to be half the man he was I'd be doing well. We shared many similarities, particularly intricate mannerisms, expressions, and catchphrases applied to common situations. "Ya beauty" and "on you go", were sentences we frequently voiced in times of jubilation, especially when it came to the successful announcement of a significant accomplishment, but more so on the golf course after sinking a match winning putt. It made me sad. He was my father, but he was my friend—maybe my best friend. It upset me more than anything that our time on the course was being cut short. There was no way I could continue walking miles around the fairways, breathing in the fresh air and the smell of freshly mowed grass. Our days of appearing in the father and son tournament were out also, and that connection during those times was eroding away at my mental state. I was just happy that my younger brother could step in and I could cheer them on to greatness, as their success would be my success. We were a family, we were one.

My mum was a sweetheart and still is to this day. She made me who I am today, and I owe her amounts of money and emotional support that could never be paid back in two lifetimes. She was a hard taskmaster, strict as hell, but kept me on the straight and narrow. She was a short lady, a real stunner in her day, dark shiny shoulder length hair, with an intellect I could only strive to match. She was about five feet two or three, but we were all short—it was a family trait. The word "wee" often preceded our first names. "Wee Brandon," "wee John," "wee Betty," and "wee Alan," my little brother—his triumphant claim to fame being he was the tallest in the family, at a towering five feet eight! My mother also wished my illness on herself. Emotionally it almost cut to the bone to know that someone would even lose both their legs if it meant you didn't have to. To have this type of support was like landing five numbers and the bonus ball in the weekly lottery. There were so many kids during high school who never even knew their father, with mother's currently under physical abuse from their current step dad, pushing them to work at the earliest of ages, void of further education in order for them to bring in some immediate money to feed their excessive drug and alcohol habits. It was sad, but unfortunately true—a feeling of neglect I fortunately would never experience.

I knew everyone meant well, but I could see in their eyes and tainted smiles that they weren't really sure that everything was going to be alright, particularly my aunt Morag. She was like a clone of my mum in every way, and just as easy to decipher. We were a close family and were there for one another, but I didn't need anyone feeling sorry for me, as it was beginning to rub off on me now! I needed to confront a Sergeant Major type, someone who would put a size twelve boot firmly up my ass and tell me to get a grip of myself and fight it with every ounce of strength I had remaining in my diminishing soul; to see the light at the end of the long, cold and damp tunnel. If there was still light, there was still a way.

I dwelled on this thought for many a sleepless night, convincing myself I was just a complaining little brat. It wasn't like I had a life threatening disease. Life altering perhaps, but the hospital during my agonizing visit had no doubt been filled with many less fortunate than me, and probably many even younger than my early adult years. Some poor little bastard would've probably bitten my hand off to receive the diagnosis. *Here, have this cancer instead you lucky twat. At least you'll likely get to see a bit the world and your own children growing up.* I could just visualize the words coming from the early teenage leukemia stricken boy, praying he'd even get to experience the horror of acne and further school yard beatings, regardless of how unpleasant they would've been—it would mean he was still alive. These thoughts were stored in the mental bank, requiring a withdrawal from the account should I fall back into my hole of self-pity.

The world was a screwed up place, nobody could doubt it. We'd sent probes to Mars, had satellites orbiting the earth, and had even discovered countless drugs to combat erectile dysfunction, but couldn't find something to completely prevent the effects of inflammation slowly eroding joint cartilage, rendering irreparable damage. I laughed as I thought of how messed up the entire pharmaceutical industry was. *Come on guys, let's focus on what really matters!* I was forced to chuckle. Viagra was a wonder drug for many, transforming their beaten and over exhausted little soldiers to immediate attention with the quick pop of a pill, providing a previously pathetic lover with the staying power of a porn star for the evening—stiff as a metal rod with negligible recovery time between sessions. The irony was comical—I was looking for a drug to relieve stiffness!

I just wanted to be treated as a normal person, was that too much to ask? My family and friends weren't doing it on purpose and obviously just wanted to help. It was the little things like insisting on opening doors for me, not letting me get a round in at the bar when it was my turn, and the worst of all, not bursting my balls the way they used to. I didn't need the oversensitivity.

They were unaware of the anguish this was causing me. I may have been less mobile than before, but mentally I was as capable as ever; essentially the same old me, and I longed to feel that way again.

Maybe I was losing my mind, but they didn't know that, and I would never tell them, but I was as smart and intellectual as ever before. I was perhaps even more knowledgeable and aware as I'd ever been. I had the time now to think of matters like never before, and had become scarily book smart.

Reading was one of the few activities I could still do with ease, and I managed to catch up on topics I'd always said I would get to, such as Scottish history and world politics. I even pulled out my French Linguaphone set that had been gathering dust on the shelf, disguising itself as an ornament for propping up my other books.

My life had definitely changed for the worse, but I didn't need the pity to reinforce my inner pain even more. Would I really be missed if I ended it all? It would be so simple to do as well. Half a pint of whiskey and a bottle of pills would easily do the trick. I'd pass out and the pain would be gone forever. Maybe there *was* an afterlife; perhaps it was one where anyone who'd suffered disease or disability was fully functional again. What if there wasn't one though? Maybe if there was, then there might be an additional punishment given out to those who took their own lives, as a result of the pain and sorrow they left their loved ones behind to deal with.

I really wanted the pain and torment to go away, but I would've essentially left my family with a pain that easily outweighed my current struggles. Ending my life would essentially be doing the same to them. If there was a heaven and we met again, how could I look them straight in the eyes and justify the torture I'd caused them for the remainder of their days on earth?

It was a selfish way out, and I had to snap myself out of this emotional hell hole that I kept falling into. My sick teenage friend was there as usual to save the day. He had a disappointed look on his face this time that almost caused me to blush.

I'm getting a little impatient by the fact we are meeting this regularly. Are you really this weak? Look at me. LOOK AT ME DAMN IT!

His stern face and furrowed brow was crystal clear in my head, and an ashamed look graced my features as I stared deep into the bathroom mirror.

Why don't you take yourself down to the Sick Children's Hospital for the afternoon? That'll give you some perspective you bloody coward. At least you have the opportunity to fight. Not me though, and not many of those sick kids either. It's too late for us. Our clock is counting down and there's no way of stopping it. The ship has sailed. You're the captain of your vessel and can decide whether it leaves the dock or not, so snap out of this cowardly self pity you weak little bastard. My parents are devastated, and I know they might never get completely over my death when it finally happens. You have a choice; not only your own fate, but the fate of those who love you. It makes me sick that you're even thinking about such a ghastly course of action!

He was right. I had to fight like a man. There was no excuse for my current thinking, and it had to stop; and that time was now.

Emotional Rollercoaster

I went back to work as usual, encountering the same pity from my co-workers as I'd received from friends and family, but I'd gotten over my initial shock, for now anyway, drifting off to the conversation with my imaginary teenage Leukemia stricken friend when I felt myself wobbling on the tightrope of depression. I wouldn't have to put up with these guys much longer anyway, as I was scheduled for hip surgery in two weeks. As I discovered though, the mind can severely alter its state in fourteen days.

Work was as strenuous as ever. I worked for a Japanese firm based in Scotland. A huge manufacturing facility that covered the area of fifty football fields—it was enormous, and fed the mouths of almost half the residents in the local area. I literally hated my manager. He was an overweight Japanese man, graying at the temples and had a head the size of a prize winning melon. His borderline obesity suited him though and was probably the only thing keeping him upright—that head must've weighed thirty pounds. His mother probably demanded a caesarian section after seeing pictures of the first scan prior to giving birth. He was growing on me though, one of the few who were almost oblivious to my pain and daily physical struggles. He was like the Sergeant Major I'd been wishing for; treating me like it was any other day or situation. I liked it as it eased my paranoia.

During coffee breaks I felt like I was attracting unwanted attention as I limped my way wearily to the cafeteria. People passed me in the corridor, saying hello, many of whom had never given me the time of day before.

I don't need your pity.

I looked forward to my major surgery, an unwanted escape route from this artificialness, but an escape route nevertheless.

I found myself breaking Japanese tradition in the few days leading up to my scheduled visit to the hospital. It was frowned upon, but I didn't care what people thought, and it seemed like I was being treated as an exception right now anyway—at least it did in my mind. It was a regimented culture, break time from 10:00—10:15am. An alarm bell sounded and we all strutted through for coffee like a troop of soldiers or coordinated marching band. Not me though. I'd sit and wait, moving sloth-like to my favorite bathroom cubicle around 10:10am, sitting in the stall, contemplating my naval. I didn't need the attention of the crowd. I'd sit there until the masses dispersed back to the open plan office, a few stragglers stopping off to pee out the over-brewed caffeine, or deposit their over indulgent quantities of Indian cuisine from the previous evening.

"How's it going Rick?" said the familiar nasally tone of Gordon Speirs—a voice as distinctive as the guy from almost every movie preview ever made.

"G'day Gordon," said Rick in his drawn out Australian twang.

Rick was my direct supervisor, one layer down from melon head, and one above the rest of us "peons." He was a health *freak*, eating nothing but soy this, soy that, and enough beans and other vegetables to clean out a produce farm in a matter of weeks. The irony was that he looked like the unhealthiest man alive, he and my present state neck and neck down the final straight. He wasn't your stereotypical Aussie. Not rough around the edges, or tough as nails, and certainly not partial to the occasional "cold one". He was tall, pale as a bottle of milk, and built like a golf club; his arms were like twigs, ready to snap as a result of a violent sneeze. He entered the cubicle next to me, door slamming and locking with an urgency of a man with only minutes to live. No sooner had the seat dropped, but the percussion began. Anyone now entering the bathroom would've wondered how an entire brass band could fit into one of the tiny stalls, vegetable tainted farts trumpeting, echoing against the walls. It was like Louis Armstrong was going all out on a stunning solo effort, blowing like the Scottish wind, cheeks expanding to their physical limit—they were in this case, but not the cheeks on Rick's face.

Finally Rick made his way out of the stall, groans of satisfaction as he dragged his scrawny ass out of the now grotesque room. As a result of the stench, I found a spurt of energy to prompt me in the direction of the canteen, the foul reek of stale broccoli and lima beans enough to pull the dead from their graves.

I sat alone with my heavily sugared coffee, chatting to the cafeteria worker by the name of Brenda. She was a weird looking woman, perhaps a couple of years my senior, not that I'd ever inquire as to the actual number. She wasn't unattractive, but her teeth were like a set of piano keys, almost Bugs Bunny like, with stereotypical ginger colored Scottish hair and an accent only recognizable to residents of the local area. Her breasts made her though, like a twin set of my Japanese manager's head, almost bursting for freedom from her less than fashionable maid-looking attire. She had a thing for me, never spoken, but I could tell. She knew I was struggling and in pain, but it seemed to boost her attraction for me, like she wanted to caress and care for me, wait on hand and foot and relieve me in ways never before encountered.

I'd occasionally arrive at work early to avoid the morning rush and associated unwanted attention. Brenda was there as usual piling on an extra sausage and rasher of bacon to my breakfast plate—defying the strict policy of the penny pinching organization. I couldn't be sure if it was because I was her favorite or if she could see my gradually reducing body mass, and felt sorry for me, her motherly instincts telling her to "do whatever it took" to fatten me up and nurse me back to fitness. Either way I was fine with it, as I knew she was genuine, favoritism or concern, an extra rasher of salty, juicy Danish bacon was never to be sniffed at.

Our office was an open plan layout; the penny pinching bastards were even too stingy to provide individual cubicles. It almost reminded me of high school physics class in the way the long desk tops were laid out, removing any possibility of privacy of any variety. I hated having to leave the main office, whether for a bathroom break or to attend a meeting in one of our plain, dreary and washed-out looking conference rooms that reminded me of the bleak Scottish weather. Every time I walked around I could sense dozens of sets of eyes, looking me up and down, scrutinizing my limping, feeling sorry for me and wondering what was *really* wrong.

Get back to work and mind your own bloody business you nosey bunch of wasters. It might give you something to gossip about at the water cooler when I'm not around, but if that's all you have to talk about, your existence is verging on being as sad as my current nightmare!

The worst moments were when it came to going down stairs—I just couldn't bring myself to do it when anyone was around. I was *so* self-conscious and would've rather swam in a piranha infested river than put on a show of pain and struggling for anyone to see. I could just see the inquiries if I made my way down like a whimpering sloth in the presence of one of my fellow smart ass colleagues. "Need a hand?" or "Is everything alright?"

No I don't need a hand, and I don't need your sympathy. As for me being alright, yes, couldn't be better! I'm having a rare old time making my way down these stairs like a crippled old aged pensioner who's taken an enormous dump in his pants!

It was a distressing thought that I was actually looking forward to the upcoming surgery. It would get me out of this place, away from all the ogling eyes and the false concern. If only they were replacing all affected joints, not just the left hip.

Make it go away, please make it go away.

Relationships

Who wanted to be tied to a man destined for an early decrepit state and perhaps wheelchair bound by the time he's forty? My girlfriend, Gillian, a stunningly beautiful twenty two year old woman openly stated she was there for me, but an intricate change in her pupil size as I told her the diagnosis didn't entirely fill me with confidence that her actions and words would go hand in hand.

We'd met—pre-diagnosis—at a local nightclub, eyes meeting from across the dance floor as she moved with the elegance of a trained dancer; her tightly toned little body moving perfectly in time with the tunes the hyperactive DJ was frantically spinning high up in his platform in the corner of the club. Her head weaved side to side, flicking her Marilyn Monroe blonde locks of hair around as they cascaded onto the silky smooth tanned shoulders that were on display as a result of the low-cut black and white striped top. During one of her mesmerizing head weaves, she caught my eye as I was stood hypnotically at the edge of the dance floor. She looked away, but there was a familiarity about me that caused her a quick double take. I gave her a wink and raised my glass of luke-warm beer in her direction, toasting her ability, but hopefully indicating my interest as well. She retorted with a seductive smile that displayed pearly white teeth that fitted like a glove with her full, glossy-looking lips that could've melted an iron bar. My pulse started to race in conjunction with my mind as I envisioned her soft naked body rubbing against mine. It was time for a *cold* beer, as my temperature was skyrocketing off the thermometer scale. As she flicked her head back to her uncoordinated friend, I made my exit in the direction of the bustling bar.

"You alright Brandon? You're looking a wee bit flustered," said my younger brother Alan as he shouted for a round of drinks to the equally flustered bartender.

"Sound wee man. Just saw a chick I kissed about two years ago. She's looking *good*. With a bit of luck I'll be in there like a dog on a pork chop."

"She got any pals?"

"She's dancing with one of them now, but she's a bit of a boiler. Nice fit body, but a face like a burst sofa."

"Not a problem to the Alan boy, why do you think they invented doggy-style. Either that or a paper bag over the head—and that's just for my noggin!"

Alan was a character. We were both pretty smooth talkers, but what I had in sophistication, he had in general goofiness and overall self-confidence. He was my "wee brother", but was two inches taller, had a better build to him and perhaps looked a year or two older, clearly defying the birth certificates that cited he was four years my junior. We were similar with our dark brown hair and certain physical features, including our facial hair which seemed to grow at an alarming rate. Those meeting us for the first time quickly concluded we were related. We were like a double act at times, often competitive, to see who could be the funniest or indeed the biggest smart ass. It was a close match, but we complimented each other well, like Laurel and Hardy without the straight man.

We stood at the bar and I pointed the girls out to Alan.

"You're right about the pal, but she's getting better with each gulp," he said, swigging eagerly from his bottle of Budweiser.

"You're a dirty wee tart. You'd stick it in a barber shop floor if there was a hole in it."

"Just trying to help my big brother out; sometimes you need to take one for the team," he said with the trusty family wink.

We could see the girls, but they couldn't see us. I was encouraged to see Gillian give an occasional glance to where I'd been previously standing—seemed the interest wasn't one-sided.

It was getting near the end of the evening, the DJ ramping down the vicious rhythm of his previous techno tunes, perhaps a result of his over exuberance of mixing and scratching of vinyl, alternating between decks like a sex starved young man encountering his first ever threesome. The music had been replaced by the usual final fifteen minutes of slow love songs, giving opportunity to those finding an evening of lust to grind against one another, with the aim of sharing a taxi ride home and hopefully breakfast. It was now or never. We moved in on the girls like a lion stalking a gazelle, tip-toe like, moving into position, ready to pounce. We had to act now, not only because the dance floor was surrounded by drunken, zombie like men looking to score, especially with Gillian, but it left enough time to potentially pick up a last minute score if we encountered rejection.

"Watch and learn brother," said Alan, moving swiftly in the direction of the ladies. He expertly caressed Burst Sofa's face, then into a waltz-like clinch, spinning her around with the ease of a trained dancer, but likely a by-product of his inebriated state and an action necessary to avoid falling flat on his drunken head. Gillian was almost in shock by the delicate maneuver, looking like a lost puppy.

She turned to leave the floor, but was stopped in her tracks by my lustful gaze. I held my palm in her direction, the words "stop right there" written all over it, as I made my way towards her, just in time, as I cut off a drunken fool with similar ideas, letting his words of "bastard" enter one ear and out the other like they'd never been uttered.

"You're very sure of yourself," she said, appearing almost objectionable, but pulling me close to her pulsating chest at the same time.

"Not really, just sure about you," I whispered in her ear, pulling my head from her shoulder and giving her a look deep into her eyes that could've melted butter.

Alan had abandoned the tender moves and was now making out with Sofa like they were a couple of washing machines on super spin cycle. All inhibition on her part had been thrown viciously out the window, and was now gripping his buttocks as though they were a couple of stress relieving balls.

"That's my brother by the way," I said to Gillian as we both laughed nervously at their antics, semi-conscious of the staring eyes around them.

"Does he take after you?" said Gillian, with an eager vibe, almost enticing me for some action.

I didn't bother to reply, replacing my prospective witty remark with a soft and tender kiss, more than appropriate for the Billy Ocean classic "Suddenly" that was barely legible in the background, being more than overpowered by the intensity of our passion.

The taxi ride home was comical. Alan a little pissed off he was riding up front with the driver, who'd obviously been working for a while with the car heater more than a fraction too high. He stunk! His appearance matched his pungent odor, stained sweatpants and a tacky looking Hawaiian shirt unbuttoned a little too far, displaying his gorilla like chest hairs that no doubt provided more insulation from the elements than any form of clothing from his nasty smelling wardrobe.

"Where we headed?" he asked with an air of confidence contrary to what I'd expected from a man of his attractiveness. I was half expecting his first line to be "the bells, the bells" such was his hunched up Quasi Modo type exterior.

"Bothwell Main Street, then onto Viewpark," I said, taking control of the situation, as Alan discreetly turned around, thumb and forefinger holding his nose, much to the amusement of Gillian and Burst Sofa, otherwise known as Angela to those close to her. We could all smell him, and were glad that home was only ten minutes away at most.

"No, we're just going to Bothwell Main Street," piped up Gillian as she tenderly rubbed my thigh. That was the location of my apartment, and my spirits rose in conjunction with the miniature tent that had instantaneously been pitched in my pants.

We left the cab with a sense of urgency, for once eager to get into the cold Scottish fresh air, and escape the fusty body odor that had terrorized our short but seemingly endless journey. I threw Quasi an extra tip, praying he'd pay a late night visit to the pharmacy for a stick of Right Guard and save the souls of his next unfortunate customers.

We entered my apartment, Alan half stumbling as he tripped on the heavily bristled welcome mat.

"Who put that there?" he said comically, over exaggerating his stagger and proceeded his way to the fridge for more alcohol. The living room was cold, contrary to the bright colors of red and blue that decorated the walls and floor, symbolic of my love for Glasgow Rangers football club, the team my wonderful father graced prior to his career ending injury.

"Bit chilly in here," stated Angela, vigorously rubbing her shoulders.

She wasn't joking, as her nipples appeared to grow before my very eyes, bullet-like and capable of hanging a couple of soaking wet coats on. Gillian wasn't far behind, but nothing in comparison to the rigid football studs that were on show from under Sofa's blouse.

"You won't be cold for long," said Alan, uncorking a bottle of cheap wine—a remnant from a previous family visit that was saved for moments of alcohol desperation, not unlike now.

"Why, you gonna turn the heating on?" replied Angela, with a look hoping he'd say no.

"Why, you lost the power of your legs? The thermostat's on the wall beside you," replied Alan, teasing her into submission.

It always amazed me how women liked a bad boy; which Alan definitely was. The way he kept them guessing, never kissing their ass, unless literally. She loved it though, and her smile couldn't be kept under wraps, no matter how hard she tried.

"That's *your* job. Not turning up the heat, keeping me warm."

The tone had been set. She would've been as well saying "take me now big boy" but Alan retained his composure.

We wolfed into the Blue Nun wine like it was a bottle of Moet Chandon, our taste buds so penetrated by the night of alcohol that it was hard to distinguish between the two. Sofa was getting restless, and mauling Alan's bottom lip like a rabid Rottweiler. His tent pole was extending with her every slurp, and I decided it was time to exit stage left.

"Wanna listen to some music in my room?" I quietly said to Gillian. It was on par with asking a woman if she'd like to come back to your place for a coffee, but far more appropriate and romantic than "fancy a shag?"

I led her eager, fit body out the living room door, almost colliding with her tight physique as she enthusiastically tried to pass me; she was obviously choking for it!

This could be a one night stand, but I treated her with the care of a bride on her wedding night, just sober enough to remember that foreplay was important as I explored her entire body. I moved over every square inch, attempting to find a blemish, but there were none to be found. Her odor was that of a flower store mixed with the exotic fruit section of the local supermarket.

There was no doubting the passion and tenderness that was on display, but it became hard to concentrate, as we both started to giggle intensely. The noises coming from Amanda and Alan next door were deafening. I had to focus hard to block out their moans and groans, but the sheer beauty of Gillian made that an easier task than I'd first imagined. There was passion between us like I'd *never* experienced before. It was like a dream that I never wanted to end.

That was then, but this was now, and the previous electricity between us was fading. It was like the electric company wasn't immediately turning out the lights, but slowly dimming them the longer the bill went unpaid, and there was a dullness appearing in my apartment during the nights Gillian and I spent together. She said it wasn't a result of my ultimate evaporating quality of life, but I knew it was. She deserved better and she knew it as well, and it wasn't long before I was back to the single life again.

Private Health Care

Surgery was tomorrow and I entered the private hospital feeling like a VIP. It was my first visit to such a venue, previously only used to the damp and dull interior of the typical National Health environment. I could feel the thick shag carpet under my feet as I checked in at the reception desk. It had more of the feel of a posh hotel than a hospital, as I half expected the cute customer friendly assistant to ask me how many nights I was planning to stay.

I was escorted to my room like I was a member of the Royal family, as the courteous, yet slightly effeminate bus boy enquired if I'd like to see a menu for dinner. *A menu for dinner!* I was only used to the school dinner variety of food that was generally presented during these visits, not hospitality of this nature.

I settled in, slightly uncomfortably, but growing more at ease as the minutes passed by. I almost forgot about the matter at hand—major surgery, such was the overwhelming nature of the visit thus far.

The nurses had a cheerfulness to them that was so refreshing compared to their National Health counterparts. There was none of the impatient attitudes, likely a result of not being rushed off their feet to quite the same degree. Public hospitals were almost like cattle markets—each ward overstocked with ill people and each room rarely occupied by only one person. These places kept your stay to a bare minimum, as vacant beds were as common as an individual lottery win. They were like production lines; as soon as a patient was checked out or indeed died, another poor bugger was dumped into the vacancy like a pile of bricks on a building site.

Not at this private establishment though. I basically had my own dedicated nurse. I believe she was looking after three patients, but it felt like she was mine, appearing like magic anytime I pressed the "call" button. She was oriental, but had lived in the UK all her life. Her name was Jenny, a softly spoken and extremely cute girl around my age. She was a tiny little thing with stereotypical straight black hair tucked up in a bun under her nurse's cap. My mind wandered as I pictured her ripping the hat off and shaking the silky hair out of its clip and flowing onto her dainty shoulders; like she would've been interested in me, with my thin frame and muscles like knots in a chicken's leg.

Stop living in a fantasy world Brandon.

"You're Surgeon will be here to see you in about an hour."

"Hope he's good at his job," I said with a chuckle.

"He's the best. He's the guy who developed the latest procedure for replacing hip replacements."

This was fantastic news and I could almost feel myself relaxing more as my head sank deeper into my pillow.

"A first time replacement should be a piece of piss to him then."

"You could put it like that," she said with a smirk.

"I'm sorry, I didn't mean to be crude, I'm just a little nervous."

"I understand Mr. Wilkinson, but you really are in the best hands here."

"Call me Brandon, please. No need for any formality when you're around me."

"OK Brandon. Well we need to get you prepared for your surgery. I'm going to have to shave the hair on your hip and the surrounding area."

"No dinner or a movie? You just want to go straight to shaving my body," I said with a wink.

"I see I've landed myself a frisky one here," she said giggling as her cheeks turned scarlet.

"I'm just messing with you."

"I can mark the area for you and you can do yourself if you'd like?"

"What, and miss out on a cute nurse doing it for me. I think not."

She laughed again and her cheeks remained cherry red. I was only half kidding. This might've been the most action I'd seen in a while and probably would be for some time as I recovered from the operation.

I lifted my gown as she headed out of the room to grab a razor and some shaving cream. The old John Thomas had seen bigger days; it wasn't cold by any means, but the entire prospect of being torn open during surgery and having a saw blade slice and dice my hip bone had probably caused the little fellow to dive into hibernation. I rubbed and pulled at his neck like a murderer throttling his cheating wife. I had to coax the little guy a bit further down the driveway than he currently was. He was no doubt going to be on display to Jenny, even though she was shaving my hip, but I wasn't wearing any underwear to act as a shield.

Jenny returned looking rather tentative. I was sure she'd had to shave many a patient before, but probably not too many of them were as cocky and flirtatious as I'd been. She carefully pulled back my gown, and as I'd thought, the old two meat and veg were on display like the last chicken hanging in a meat cupboard. Fortunately my efforts of reviving a bit of life into the little chap had been a complete success and I wasn't as self conscious as I might have been. Her touch on my outer thigh was soft and smooth as she applied the shaving cream, and I resisted all temptation to make any wise cracks. It was strangely erotic, so I filled my mind with thoughts of soccer games, wrinkly old people, and generally anything that could avoid springing the little man to a sudden upright position.

Jenny made her way to tend to another patient and I lay playing the shaving experience over in my head. As I looked around, I still couldn't get over the plush interior of the room. It really was on par with the Hilton hotel I'd spent a couple of nights in a few years back. The TV was equipped with satellite channels, not just your terrestrial five channels that were part of the basic set-up. I had Sky sports and news, as well as Euro Sport, a luxury I didn't even have at home. The décor was fantastic also; peaceful looking landscapes were framed on the walls, adding to the overall comfort of the place, perhaps these pictures were deliberately chosen to give the patients a feeling of being one with nature and relax them even more prior to any surgical procedure. The towels in the bathroom were as thick as quilts and there was even a chunky looking bathrobe hanging on the door. I chuckled, wondering how I was going to get my bag zipped up when I was due to leave.

One of the landscaped paintings on the wall was of a peaceful lake surrounded by what appeared to be the tranquil hills of the Scottish countryside; a few distant sheep on the slopes being the only sign of life. I gradually dozed off, visualizing myself on a boat out there, breathing in the calm fresh air and not having a worry in the world. My eyes suddenly opened to find myself on the operating table as the saw blade hacked its way through my hip bone. The pain was unbearable as I screamed in tune with the surgeons laughter, and small fragments of bone flew in succession towards my face like bullets from a machine gun.

"Aahhhhhhh," I yelled, sitting abruptly upright.

"Mr. Wilkinson, it's alright."

"What the hell."

"You were just dreaming Mr. Wilkinson."

I grasped at my hip. It *had* just been a nightmare as everything was intact; but it was a visualization that was now going to increase my fear when the actual procedure was due to take place.

Standing in front of me were Jenny and the guy who'd just spoken to me. He was in his early fifties, and smartly dressed—if somewhat old-fashioned looking—in a brown plaid sports jacket with matching tie and white shirt.

"Brandon, this is Mr. Ivory, he'll be the one performing your surgery," said Jenny, looking a little disturbed by my outburst.

"Hi Mr. Ivory; I apologize for that, I was just having a bit of a nightmare about the procedure. I won't go into detail about it as you'll probably think I'm completely nuts," I said with a smile.

"That's OK Mr. Wilkinson; it's often a common occurrence for people going through major surgery. Mental anxiety regularly triggers these types of dreams."

He had an extremely calm demeanor to his voice; the type of tone you'd find from the narrator of a relaxation tape. I was also encouraged by his title of "Mister." In the medical field this was actually a step above the level of Doctor.

"Cool, glad to hear it's not just me, but still a little embarrassing all the same."

"It's not the first time I've seen it happen and I'm certain it won't be the last. Anyway, although your surgery is technically classed as major, I've lost count the number of times I've performed the procedure, and they've *always* been successful. I've also carried out several replacements of replacements in the last month, and those are considerably more complicated, and I haven't had any glitches there either, so just relax, I'll make you all better."

His air of confidence was unprecedented, yet delivered in such a genuine tone and void of any boasting or smugness.

"Thanks Mr. Ivory, I really needed to hear that. I know it's probably routine for you, but I've never gone through anything like this before."

"You'll be good as new tomorrow and will be wondering what all the fuss was about," he smiled, as did Jenny.

They carefully wheeled me in my bed towards the operating theatre. I nervously smiled at the patients and staff we passed in the hallway, and I could see them wondering what I was in here for and where I was headed.

"Good luck," said an elderly gentleman yielding a metal walker.

I didn't want luck to play a part in this. Luck in my book was reserved for a game of bingo or finding a parking spot at the mall on a busy Saturday afternoon, not when you were about to have your leg ripped open and permanently restructured.

We entered the operating theatre; the hospital workers using the end of the bed like a battering ram to burst open the double swing doors.

"How you feeling Mr. Wilkinson?" said Mr. Ivory, all gowned up and ready to go.

"A little anxious to say the least, but just glad there's some light at the end of the tunnel for me."

"You'll be just fine. We'll be done in about an hour and a half. You'll wake up as good as new, back in the comfort of your room. This is Dr. Gow, he's your anesthesiologist. He'll be the one who's going to send you into a wonderful dream."

"Hi there Dr. Gow. Make sure you don't penny pinch on the drugs," I said with a wink.

"Hi Mr. Wilkinson. Don't worry about that, I've been doing this a while and have the precise dose calculated. I'll have you asleep in just a few minutes."

He held a prepared syringe up and moved it towards the large vein on the back of my right hand.

"OK, this may sting a little."

It did a little, but I was so used to being jagged by needles that it didn't faze me. As he pushed in the liquid content though, the burning sensation was incredible as I could feel it work its way down the vein and into my system.

"I see what you mean about the sting now," I said, giving him a stare, and he gave me a chuckle.

"This is the point I feel like a hypnotist. You're feeling very sleepy," he replied in a put on deep voice.

He wasn't kidding either. My eyelids were becoming as heavy as rocks and the more I tried to fight it, the heavier they became. My vision was blurring and the previous bare surroundings of the operating room turned into one huge white haze.

Recuperation

The effect of removing a screwed up joint and replacing it with a titanium version was astounding. My hip was a little stiff to move but there was no pain anymore, which had previously been linked together like a couple of Siamese twins. The most pain in that area was from the wound where they had ripped me apart like a pack of wild dogs, but it was mediocre compared to the acute joint pain from before, so I treated it like a minor irritation.

I lay back in confusion in my hospital bed, following a fly around as it buzzed and meandered across the ceiling. The last thing I remembered was the anesthetic being administered and my eyes slowly closing.

"How you feeling Brandon?" said nurse Jenny, entering the room in a very upbeat manner.

"Hey Jenny, feeling much better thanks; still feeling a little groggy, but the hip joint pain has gone. It's sore on the side of the leg, but I think that's just from where they cut me open."

"That's wonderful. You'll need to spend the next day in bed, but after that we'll have you up walking around."

Wow, there was no messing about; I loved it.

"We've hooked you up to some IV medication, if the pain from the operation gets a little much, just press the attached button.

"Great, I shouldn't need it, but thanks."

I didn't really need it, but after I was told it was a liquid form of Morphene, I changed my tune.

As soon as Jenny left the room, I pushed the button to administer some of the drug. About ten minutes later there was a calmness about me that felt *so* good. It was as though I didn't have a care in the world. It was like a mixture of being stoned and having a small alcohol buzz. I was just glad I was lying down as my legs tingled, and I wasn't sure they would've supported my weight even if I'd wanted them to.

Jenny popped her head around the door.

"A couple of visitors are here to see you."

"Hey, company, who is it?" I said in a mellow sounding tone straight out of a Cheech and Chong movie.

"Alright son," said my Dad, looking extremely happy. I was sure Jenny had already informed him that the operation had been a complete success, as I knew he'd been more worried than I was prior to the surgery.

"Hey Dad, how's it going?"

"Much better now."

"Hey Scott."

My buddy Scott was there as well, and he was grinning from ear to ear.

"You still high on the drugs they gave you? You look well wasted."

"Not at all; I was a little groggy after the operation, but they gave me this liquid Morphene stuff to ease the pain. I don't think I need it, but figured as it was legal in here as well as being free, it would've been virtually criminal not to give it a try."

They both laughed emphatically as they shook their heads. I was sure if it had been under any other circumstances they would've given me a hard time, but not today. They were both concerned about me and just delighted that everything had gone to plan and things were looking brighter for me.

After telling them I loved them—due to my mashed up state—I told them of the episode of Jenny shaving me in preparation for the operation. They got a major kick out of that as I could tell they thought Jenny was a cute one, but they also they seemed over the moon that my spirits were so high.

"They said they'll have me up and walking around tomorrow."

"Really?" said my Dad, somewhat in disbelief.

"Yeah, that's what they said. I'll still have to use the crutches, but they want me to start putting weight on it as soon as possible. Then in a week or so they've scheduled some hydrotherapy. Think they want to do it in water as it has less of an impact to the joints or something."

"That's great, pal. Son, it's really great to see you so upbeat. We've all been really worried about you for a while. You've just seemed so down."

"I know Dad, it's been really rough. I'm sorry about the moods and stuff, but I've been having a hard time getting my head around all this. I always thought arthritis was an old person's disease, and it's been hard getting my head around the idea that I won't be able to do martial arts ever again, as well as soccer and just about anything that requires running around. I feel bad about it, as things really could be a lot worse. I've been thinking a lot about all these young kids in the world with terminal conditions who would give their right arm to be in my position. Those thoughts have really put this into a whole new perspective for me."

Scott and my Dad were silent for a few seconds, and I could almost see their eyes filling up a little. It was a true statement to make though and I had to keep that in mind, particularly in the tough times that no doubt lay ahead.

After my Dad and Scott had left, I gave myself another hit of the Morphene and slid down the bed from my sitting position and sank the back of my head into the soft feathered pillow. My mind was working overtime, but I was becoming sleepier by the second. The recovery was going to be difficult, but I was determined to put in the required effort to maximize the benefits from the surgery.

"Good morning Mr. Wilkinson."

My eyes opened wearily, but squinted immediately as the sunlight from the window instantly connected with them.

"Good morning?"

"Yes, good morning. I hear you had quite a sleep last night," said Mr. Ivory, looking rather amused.

"Holy crap, it must've been. It was early evening the last I remember."

"Well you went through quite an ordeal yesterday, so it's not uncommon to be exhausted."

"Wow, you don't say; I haven't slept that good in a long time."

"How are you feeling?"

"Pretty good Mr. Ivory," I said, finally getting my bearings. "The wound is a little tender, but the hip pain has gone. It feels a little stiff, but getting rid of the pain is the main thing."

"That's fantastic. Well I just want to let you know that the operation went great and I'm really happy with it. Jenny will be through to see you shortly. I want you up on your feet this morning to get the hip moving. She will take you through a few exercises, but you'll find that the stiffness should subside in a couple of days. Just get some breakfast in you first to get a little energy then you'll be ready to start your recuperation."

"Mr. Ivory, I can't thank you enough and I don't know if I'll ever be able to repay you properly."

"Don't be silly, I'm just doing my job. If I know you're feeling better and you get the functionality back in your hip that is more than enough repayment for me."

I was becoming a little emotional. This guy was *so* genuine and I could sense his sincerity. He was a good man, who obviously got a lot of job satisfaction from improving the quality of life for his patients.

"Thank you sir, you have no idea what this means to me though."

"I think I do. Just promise me that you'll give the physical therapy all the effort you have. It will be a long journey ahead for you, but you're young and will be able to recover much quicker than most of my older patients."

"You got my promise."

"Best of luck today Mr. Wilkinson; I'll be back to see you tomorrow."

They discharged me from the hospital with an array of items designed to assist me over the coming weeks. There were crutches, a raised toilet seat, another high seat with four legs that could be put into the shower so I didn't have to stand and risk slipping on the wet tile, and also a bottle of fluid for cleaning my lovely new wound!

The raised toilet seat was about ten inches thick and fitted on top of my existing one. It was so I didn't strain too much and make it easier getting back to my feet after doing my business. It was a weird view from this location, like actually sitting on a throne, and gave me a great insight into what it must be like for Shaquille O'Neil to take a number two, with the exception that my feet dangled about six inches above the small black rug that fit snuggly around the base of the toilet like the neck of a t-shirt.

Even with the other seat that fitted conveniently into the shower, getting in and out was a delicate and potentially dangerous process, and I was extremely cautious when I washed, as my hip was feeling great and I didn't want to risk damaging it already and requiring further surgery.

The contraption for the shower had two plastic arms on it like a cheap office chair, and each of the four legs had a rubber stopper at the ends to give some adhesion and prevent slippage, but without actually screwing the legs down to the floor, there was always an element of maneuverability, usually at the most inopportune moment. I would delicately climb into the shower. The hardest part was discarding my crutches and transitioning to the shower seat. My paranoia would kick in at this time, and if anything I was even over precautious, a habit that I didn't perceive as being a bad one.

The first time I sat in the shower, I wondered if the exact same apparatus was provided to those over the age of sixty-five. Were the plungers on the seat legs replaced by four tennis balls like they used on their walkers? Probably not, but the idea made me chuckle. We could send men to the moon, fly a laser guided missile through the front door of a home in another country, but hadn't come up with something more technologically advanced for grip purposes on the feet of a metal walker. It's a sad day when renewing some of the accessories on these pieces of equipment required a visit to Sports Authority!

Recovery was tough, but I had the determination of a starving Pit Bull. My spirits were higher than usual as a result of the eradicated hip pain. Pre-op it had been wildly hindering me; every step onto my left leg sent a pain surge with the intensity of a lightening bolt, all the way from the affected joint and down to my toes.

My overall pain may have dulled, but my tiredness was compensating for this. The physical therapy, light stretching, and other hip mobility exercises were kicking the crap out of me. I had a new surge of energy, but my body was no longer acclimated to deal with such a level of activity.

Come on kid, keep it going.

It was tough, but hopefully all worthwhile. Nobody could tell for sure, but of all the factors that could taint possible success, lack of effort and determination would not be one of them.

Hope

The hip felt wonderful, and the pain from the huge incision had almost gone, with the black and blue bruising around the stitches now going through its yellow jaundice phase.

It was going to leave an almighty scar, but the story possibilities were virtually endless; not that it was likely that I'd have my naked upper thigh and hip area on display to any female companion—but I could fantasize.

Maybe I'd tell them a small five foot reef shark briefly grabbed me when I was swimming off the east coast of Florida. "And this one time … at Daytona Beach." Either that or I'd been charging down a slide at a water park and unknown to me some sadistic hooligan had stuck a razor blade to the side of the tube with a piece of chewing gum. That might get a nice little bit of sympathy attention. Or I could just grow a pair of gonads and tell the real story, but it just wasn't as sexy and macho sounding as the razor or mini Jaws versions.

The hydrotherapy was really helping my other joints as well, but my right knee still suffered between sessions as a result of my bad habit of favoring that side. It was a confidence thing. Mr. Ivory had told me that the special cement used on the new hip was strong enough to support a four hundred pound man, but it was still a subconscious notion to protect it a little.

Was this the foundation of a new beginning? Was there finally some hope peering above the peak of the arthritis mountain? Who really knew? It may only be a new start for my hip, but it was at least something. You had to start somewhere. Even if this only helped my fragile mind, it could potentially have a knock on effect to my entire life.

The rehabilitation continued on for a couple of months, but my struggles reemerged. The fake joint was great, but the stark realization was that the only way the other joints would have long term relief would be to have them also turned from bone and cartilage into titanium and super strength adhesive!

South of the Border

I'd been unhappy with my current job for quite some time. It wasn't even a consequence of my negative attitude resulting from the disease. The people were fine in small doses, the general workers that was, but the management were a bunch of useless idiots who never listened to the inputs we provided them with as far as making improvements to our products. They were all middle aged Japanese men, set in their ways and had been sent over to Scotland to manage the new facility that had been purchased in their efforts to break into the European market. My melon headed boss was one of the worst—an opinion on everything, master of nothing. A manager in my mind was someone who could make decisions, take information on board, process it using knowledge of business operations, and decide whether to pursue it or not or at least ask some relevant questions requesting further information. Every one of these steps was never part of his judgment methodology. He would call our headquarters in Tokyo or a sister plant in Hiroshima or Kumamoto and see if the idea was something that was currently in place in Japan. If yes, the idea was seen as a stroke of genius and given full support with the implementation process. If no, it was immediately shot down in flames without further discussion.

Japanese culture baffled me. There was such a respect hierarchy that in my opinion added so many layers of red tape to daily business that it in fact resulted in much inefficiency and missed opportunity. It had been playing on my mind for some time as suggestion after suggestion was dismissed. "If it's not currently done in Japan there's no need to bother" seemed to be the attitude. Many coworkers felt the same, as the disappointments gradually chipped away at our overall morale. We were a group of experienced professionals within our field, knowledge vastly exceeding Honeydew Heid's capabilities.

It had been three months since the hip surgery, and I was feeling a lot better. I was still riddled with pain in most joints, but I was pain free in the one that had been causing me some of the most unbearable moments.

We had a large visit scheduled today from one of our key customers that included in depth auditing of our manufacturing and test processes. Two weeks previously I'd submitted a finely detailed action plan for some of the key areas we should examine based on current performance metrics. I even listed some of the analysis tools and techniques that should be applied and documented, and these studies could be used as excellent objective evidence to show the German customer, Bosch, who were visiting. As usual Heid-san digested the plan, closely followed by picking up the telephone receiver and pressing number one on his speed dial. It was probably labeled "decision button"!

I returned back to my desk as he rambled on at a hundred miles an hour in Japanese. It was comical the way they bowed, even when on the telephone. I'd seen it many times in person; the more senior the person, the more pronounced the bow would be. He must've really been yapping to a top level guy. He was bowing every other word, resembling something from a Japanese workout video. At one point I was extremely worried for his computer monitor as he gave an almighty bow and nearly smashed his noggin straight into it—which would obviously have been the end of that piece of hardware. I chuckled to myself as he continued on with his ass kissing. Maybe the Japanese military had signed him up to donate his head to future weapon development programs. Holy crap, if the Americans had dropped his skull from a plane, Hiroshima would still be under reconstruction.

Finally his call was over, and he sat expressionless as usual, not even gesturing for me to come to his desk. I approached anyway and stood there for what seemed like ten minutes. He didn't even raise his eyes to acknowledge my existence. Maybe he couldn't. Perhaps his neck muscles had finally just given up. Wishful thinking on my part; he was just an ignoramus. I cleared my throat and finally he registered me.

"So should I begin implementing the plan now and have everything in place for the customer visit?" I tentatively asked.

"No need. Not necessary. Japan say not required," he said in his blunt regimental tone, before refocusing on the report he was reading when I'd approached him.

That was that, a big fat waste of time on my part. I'd really poured my heart and soul into that proposal and I knew it was good. I wanted to ask Heid what *he* thought.

"Screw Japan for a minute! Even tell me OFF THE RECORD what you think, and then go stick your crotch in some fertilizer and grow some balls!"

That's what I wanted to say, but I had a mortgage and car payment to make, so it wasn't a good time to be fired.

Our German customers arrived. Three men and one woman, all dressed extremely well, carrying very official looking brown leather briefcases. They all appeared very stern and straight laced, and probably hadn't had a good laugh since they popped out of their mothers. It wasn't a country renowned for its endless comedy creations.

We congregated in the boardroom; a plush looking venue filled with a huge oval style table surrounded with mahogany carved chairs and walls decorated with pictures of the company's rise from building foundations to the impressive structure it was today. Our German customers were all business though and took no notice of the history, preferring to take their spots at the head of the table. It was standing room only, and I was one of the unfortunate ones in light of my middle of the road position within the organization. The meeting hadn't even commenced, but I was nervous already.

Our Senior Leadership Team, or SLT as they were referred to (they just had to have an acronym for everything!), gave the seemingly uninterested Germans a presentation on our financial performance and key factory processes. This was as much corporate propaganda rather than a genuine attempt to impress. It was a scheduled two day visit, and the overly detailed slide show was more of a stalling tactic; the more time spent in the boardroom, the less time our customers would have on the shop floor delving into our mediocre production lines.

The boardroom was aptly named; most people looking as though they were being made to watch a documentary on the soothing affects of watching paint dry! Personally I was losing the will to breathe, but tried to appear interested, as the eyes of our Human Resources Manager, Matt Jacobs, eagerly scanned the room, probably just looking for any excuse to call someone to his office after the meeting to rant on about professionalism during critical customer visits. Every time I sensed his wandering eyes burning a hole in the side of my head, I would give a little nod towards the presenter as though I was intrigued and agreeing with their statements.

Matt was such a douche bag. I'd heard many a story about his behavior out of office hours. The late night drinking, womanizing, not to mention slating every company policy we had ever implemented. He was such a hypocrite as he delivered speeches wearing his imaginary corporate "cap" at Town Hall meetings, stressing the importance of our ethics policies and procedures; beyond the office environment he was likely one of the greatest offenders.

It was the turn of our customers to say a few words. The tall, fair haired, yet slightly balding gentleman stood up abruptly, almost at attention. I figured from his immaculate posture that he'd probably spent some time in the German armed forces. He had a pair of silver framed John Lennon style glasses that actually looked well at home on his long pointed nose. Throw a long knee length black leather jacket over his shoulders and he could've doubled as a former member of the Gestapo. He addressed us with the sternness of such a secret police operative grilling the accused.

"Vot vee vont to see eez zee actual operation of your factory. Vee vant to see now. Vee do not need enzee more of zeez dull presentations."

This guy was not pulling any punches, and there was an almost eeriness encompassing the room right now, many of us not knowing where to look. I had to admire the Germans though, they were straight to the point, no messing around, and certainly weren't flawed with the corporate spin doctoring that was spread through Western society like an epidemic. This no-nonsense approach could only assist an organization in becoming more efficient and profitable. As long as people were allowed to make mistakes at times and not punished if they were open about them, then it could definitely work. I wasn't sure if this was completely the case in German society, but I was sure it wasn't as full of bullshit artists like many British and US companies certainly were.

In a way I felt sorry for many corporate CEO's in Western countries. Not too sorry in light of their million dollar plus annual salaries, but more because of the difficultly of their tasks. A decision is only as good as the information that goes into making it, and for large corporations this is a hurdle that is often impossible to jump. By the time a potential screw-up clambers its way up the hierarchical beanstalk, the piece of crap can often doctor its way into a candy coated golden nugget; but in today's blame culture this was a hard issue to resolve.

We were set to reconvene our meeting in four hours, and I knew we were in trouble. I was aware of the solutions to the problems that would no doubt arise. These folks seemed meticulous by nature, and if they were as knowledgeable as they came across, they would be all over some of our fundamental shortcomings that were sitting there like a group of haystacks in a pile of needles.

They were the same issues I'd raised recently to my manager who was missing a pair. He could've supported my initiative long before, and although I may have ended up having the satisfaction of saying "I told you so," I was now feeling very unsatisfied in my job role due to the lack of influence I had, and the overall value I *wasn't* adding to the company.

We gathered again in the "bored" room at 4:00 pm; our overseas colleagues looking even less jovial than they had been earlier, which was a tremendous achievement by itself.

Again the Hitler type gentleman took the floor to present their findings.

"Vee are very concerned vith many of your operations, vich in our opinion are extremely fundamental problems zat do not provide us with much confidence that you can meet our requirements in order for us to offer you our business."

He harped on for about fifteen minutes, addressing us like a school teacher scolding a classroom of delinquent students. Not once did Heid-san look in my direction, but I knew he knew he could've avoided this lecture had he followed my earlier recommendation and project plan. He would never admit that though.

The end of the day finally arrived, and I limped like a wounded soldier back to my desk; so now my physical appearance matched the emotional beating we'd all just received. I had been right all along as Adolf had detailed some of the improvement steps we needed to implement before we would be able to satisfy their needs; all of which I had clearly documented on my previous suggestion. This only fed my growing feelings of job dissatisfaction.

I logged into my computer and immediately began adding a few finishing touches to my resume. It was pretty much up to date as I knew my decision for a career change was nearing the end of the plank, but today it was finally time to jump ship.

"Hello, could I speak to a Mr. Brandon Wilkinson please?"

"Speaking."

"Hi Mr. Wilkinson, this is David Stevenson from Diamond Recruitment. Is now a good time to discuss a few potential job opportunities?"

It had only been two days since I'd submitted my resume to the recruiter, but my downbeat demeanor was promptly lifted after he'd introduced himself.

"Absolutely David," I replied with a cheerful ring to my voice.

"Sounds like I caught you on a good day."

"It might be, but I'll let you know at the end of the call," I said in my upbeat tone.

"Great. Well I got your resume and matched it with a couple of suitable openings on our system. There is one with a major corporation that I think might be of particular interest to you. It is a program management role within their Quality department, reporting to the Senior Manager. It is a full-time position that is offering a rather impressive annual salary, private medical benefits, as well as a bonus structure based around the business performance. Does this sound like something that may be of interest to you?"

It was like music to my ears. Like any job description though, they are often dressed up in fine clothes, perfect hair and make-up, and sexy sounding voice, only to discover you'd landed an old troll after the real appearance rears its head; generally when it's too late.

"It definitely *sounds* just what I'm looking for, so I am more than interested."

"Perfect. Well if you don't mind I'd like to call the recruitment person in their HR department and send over a copy of your resume and I'll get back to you as soon as I hear anything."

"Sounds great David; thanks for the call, it certainly brightened up my day."

"No problem Mr. Wilkinson, have a good day."

It had been a typically uninspiring morning until that point, but I was then filled with hope that there was perhaps a way to free myself from this corporate prison.

Inversely proportional to my mood, my work rate that afternoon was on a freefall. The reports I had to complete could wait until tomorrow as I was certainly in no rush, as being productive was the last thing on my mind. Who was going to pay attention to any further business improvement recommendations anyway, especially with my nutless manager at the top of the distribution list?

Suddenly my phone rang.

"Mr. Wilkinson?"

"David Stevenson, how are you? I didn't expect a call from you quite so soon."

I recognized his voice immediately. He was obviously from Liverpool originally, and he sounded like an absolute ringer for one of The Beatles.

"Great news for you. I spoke with the HR lady and they'd like to fly you down for an interview."

"Fly me down!"

"Yeah, turns out the position is based at their Swindon facility; about sixty miles West of London."

"Wow, I was really looking for a new job, but hadn't considered the possibility of leaving Scotland."

"Oh, OK; would you like me to tell them you're not interested?"

"No, not at all, you just caught me a wee bit off guard. No, go ahead and set something up; no harm in at least talking to them. It's not like I have any relationship ties here holding me back."

"No worries. I'll touch base with them again and let you know ASAP."

"David, thanks for your help with this."

"Not a problem; talk soon."

I mulled over the idea for a few moments and it started to grow on me. A new start in a new country might be just what I needed. It wasn't like it was in Australia or anything. My only concern was being away from my family and friends, but it would only be about a five or six hour drive away. The major fear was how I would cope with my illness if I only had myself as support on a daily basis. Perhaps this was the Sergeant Major solution that would put a size twelve boot up my ass. It would force me to be tough, fend for myself at all times, and prevent any laziness that often resulted on my part as I knew I had folks here to assist or happily perform tasks for me if I felt a little sore or just plainly couldn't be bothered.

David got back to me with the interview date. It was the following Monday. I'd fly down, all expenses paid on the Sunday evening to London Heathrow, taxi over to the hotel, full day of interviews in the morning, before catching the night flight back to Scotland on the Monday evening. I was excited about it, and although my parents were happy for me, they were extremely worried about the potential of me having to look after myself, morning, noon, and night.

"Mum, I'd be fine. It might be the best thing for me. It'll force me to be a little more independent. I wouldn't have much to do at nights, so I could focus on my stretching and exercises. I'll be as limber as a gymnast before you know it."

I laughed, and a glimmer of hope appeared in her eyes. She was obviously heartened by my level of optimism and determination, and probably believed the words more than I did myself. Of course, I didn't have the job yet, so we were all getting a little ahead of ourselves, but if an offer was given, it was one I figured would be worth taking a gamble on.

It was a typically grey, cold, and rainy Scottish afternoon as my Mum drove me to Glasgow airport. It was a Sunday, so unlike normal midweek chaos, traffic on the Kingston Bridge that spanned the river Clyde was light and flowing well. I loved looking out over the river that segregated the North and South side of the city. It was a beautiful town, but had seen many changes since I was a small boy. The area around the river used to be a huge ship building, working class area, bustling with tradesmen performing an honest day's graft. These days though had a more upscale feel to it. The river was now lined with yuppy style apartment buildings charging ridiculous monthly rent due to the prime location. The previous shipyard area now replaced with a modern exhibition center used for business conferences and rock concerts, and another building known as the "Armadillo" due to the modern shape of the structure that resembled the armored shell of the distant cousin of the anteater.

We finally approached the airport. I loved planes, and found it fascinating how such large and heavy passenger vehicles were engineered to glide in for a landing with the grace of an eagle. I used to adore flying as well, but hated it now. The cabin was like a torture chamber for my body. By the time the little "ping" noise chimed at the end of the flight, signifying safe seatbelt removal, I was so stiff it was like someone had welded me to the chair. On a long flight I'd try to get up and hobble around, but there wasn't much room to stretch out. I always got an aisle seat to at least give me the option of moving around without bothering anyone sitting next to me, but the passageway was barely wide enough for the flight attendants' cart never mind anything else; I was always being hit by those things. Even if my arm was hanging over the edge of the armrest by about the width of a pubic hair, the effeminate steward always managed to crack me on the elbow on the way past, without even the most girly of acknowledgments.

The only other area for possible stretching relief was the bathroom; but there was hardly enough room in there to take a crap, so a few light lunges were out of the question. People who bragged about how they were members of the exclusive mile high club must've really been closet contortionists; unless they'd really been on their own and claiming masturbation on a technicality.

Fortunately this trip was an extremely short one; forty four minutes to be precise—according to my ticket. The flight path must've been like an isosceles triangle; heading up at forty-five degrees, zero pause at maximum height, then descending down at the same angle, straight to the terminal building.

"That won't give you much time if you want to make it into my exclusive club," said my buddy Chris earlier that morning.

"Dude, forty-four minutes is plenty. I don't need to do it twenty-two times you know. Once would be more than adequate," was the only smart-ass reply I could muster. To this day though, I really believe he was one of the folks claiming a solo flight as satisfying the membership requirement!

My mother insisted on lifting my overnight bag from the trunk.

"I can get it!"

"I know you can son, but it's no big deal."

She gave me a tighter hug than usual and I headed into the check-in desk. I'd never let her know, but I was glad of the assistance with the luggage, as I was as stiff as a plank of wood and the pain was shooting through me, even from the short twenty five minute journey.

The check-in area was quiet for a change; probably a result of most of the London business travelers catching the Monday morning red-eye.

I was thin and gaunt looking, and my slow and deliberate limping steps were cause for a sorry tale. I caught the eye of the make-up caked desk lady from several steps away, and it seemed like an eternity before I eventually made it to the counter, enough time for her to be feeling sorry for me as I could see the concerned look on her face.

"Hi sir, how are you today?" she chirped in a cheerful rhythmical tone.

"I've been better," I said with a grimace.

"I can tell; you look like you're in a bit of pain."

"Yes I am; had an operation on my knees. They should be a bit better in a few weeks."

"Well good luck with that. Where are you flying to this afternoon?"

"Heathrow," I said, handing her my ticket.

I often made up the excuse of a knee operation. It just made things easier to explain to people I was only interacting with for a few minutes, and deflected any further unwanted pity that would've resulted from revealing the truth.

"Have a nice flight Mr. Wilkinson," she said with the customary smile as she handed me my boarding pass.

I returned a forced smile as I was aching all over and knew it was going to be quite a walk by the time I made it through security until arrival at the departure gate.

The security experience in the UK was a much friendlier one than what I'd previously encountered in the USA. For one, they actually didn't view the average Joe as a potential criminal or terrorist, and secondly, you weren't required to remove your shoes or laptop computer from its carry case—stating the screening technology was good enough to make those tasks redundant. The workers didn't have the arrogant attitudes of their US counterparts that seemed to go hand in hand with the feeling of law enforcement empowerment that occurred as soon as they pulled on their security uniform.

I finally arrived at the departure gate, literally exhausted. Typically the horizontal conveyor belts aimed at helping you on your way with limited effort had not been operational for whatever reason and my initial hope of taking a much needed rest while still making forward progress received a firm kick to the nuts.

I sipped on a piping hot, grossly overpriced cup of coffee as I waited for the flight to be called. They really should've had the cafeteria workers clothed in Dick Turpin outfits, as handing over a small fortune equivalent to the weekly wage of a Chinese factory operator was highway robbery to say the least.

The flight was eventually called, and I sat patiently as the business class passengers smugly made their way down the ramp to take their positions in their plush roomy seats and prepare themselves for the complimentary champagne prior to take-off; a luxury us coach class folks were not privileged to.

After a short time the remainder of us in the lounge was summoned. We slowly shuffled our way down to the aircraft like the cattle we were. The short trip down the enclosed corridor was agonizing. We were moving at a snail's pace in between the series of stops and starts. I wished I'd been wearing my leather jacket or any form of coat for that matter, as I could feel the cold and damp air chilling me to the bones as it leaked its way through the fine gaps in the walls of the constructed passageway.

I'd been on many a plane ride, and it was always a slow process before you could take your seat. A bottleneck always reared its ugly head, usually a result of some inconsiderate idiot who was too lazy to check in an oversized bag, deciding instead to bring it as hand luggage, trying intensely to cram it into the tight overhead compartment like a two year old frantically attempting to push his square building block into the round hole. Why security didn't force these folks to check-in such bags was beyond me.

I made my way up the aisle towards my seat, after having George the air steward quickly look at my boarding pass and tell me my chair was about halfway up on the right hand side. Why they felt the need to provide directions baffled me. What was I going to do, take a wrong turn?

To my delight the center and window seat was already occupied. I hated getting situated and then having to get up again. Beside me were two business suit types, already chatting about stocks and shares; a subject matter I had little knowledge of and even less interest in. The guy in the middle was obviously no stranger to a cheeseburger, and the buttons on his blue silk shirt looked as though they were fighting the possibility of being projected into the seats three rows in front each time he gave a hearty chuckle to his attentive new friend. The guy window side was balding on top, but had a strategic comb-over to convince everyone otherwise, but it was as believable as throwing a pair of glasses on Christopher Reeves and telling us he wasn't actually Superman.

They continued whittling on with their high finance chit-chat and I sat down. They seemed almost oblivious to my presence, which suited me fine. The aircraft engine was already fired up, and I listened intently for the sound of any unwanted rattle that could've had me on edge. Fortunately all seemed to be in order, so I relaxed completely, wishing I was part of the Champagne club in the business class section.

"Ladies and gentlemen; we will now be playing a short safety instructional video. If we could have your attention during this time it would be greatly appreciated," said the polite, sweet sounding voice of Mandy, the long-legged model-type stewardess, as the little individual TVs for each row flipped open.

I could understand why they showed the safety videos, as far as covering themselves from a legal perspective, but to call them a waste of time was an understatement. For starters, if you couldn't figure out the seatbelt procedure on your own, you should lose all entitlement of being allowed to step onto an airplane again. The only folks being attentive to that part of the film were probably the excess baggage idiots attempting to squeeze their square pegs into the round holes.

The crash position explanation always cracked me up as well. If we were heading towards the ground like a javelin, the last thing on my mind would be to remain seated, belt fastened, hunched over with my head on my knees. My first priority with certain death as the likely outcome, regardless of the position I located myself in, would be to proposition the leggy Mandy or any female with a pulse for that matter, and see if they wanted to act out any sexual fantasy they had on their "do before I die" list.

The only sensible part of the safety video in my opinion was with regard to the oxygen mask; but even having everyone adhere to that process would be a stretch to say the least. I didn't have any young children of my own, but if that day ever came around I was damn sure I wouldn't be taking time to ensure my own mask was secure prior to tending to my kids.

The safety procedure torture was finally over and the little TV screens flipped back up with their mechanical sounding buzz, and it was the Captain's turn to have a word.

"Ladies and gentlemen, this is your Captain speaking. We have a couple of aircraft ahead of us on the take-off schedule, but I'll have us up and out of here as soon as air traffic control gives us the go ahead. Our flight time today will be approximately forty five minutes and the current conditions at Heathrow are dry and overcast, with a temperature of sixty-eight degrees. So just relax and we'll do everything we can to make your flight a pleasant one. Our staff will be around about ten minutes after take-off to offer you some refreshments."

The Captain just *sounded* like he was tall, good-looking, with a chiseled, square-shaped jaw structure. He had the stereotypical posh English accent; no doubt a result of attending one of the top private schools in the South East.

We were ready for take-off, and Mandy worked her way down the aisle making sure everyone was buckled up as required and had their seat in an upright position. Part of me believed that the belt check was an excuse for them to have a sneaky crotch inspection; a suspicion that was further enhanced as George came by for a prolonged look. Was Mandy's check not good enough? I'd been tempted to roll-up the in flight magazine and slip it down my pants on the inside of the thigh. That might give them something to talk about, and perhaps be the best use the publication had ever encountered, as it was generally filled with useless advertisements and pointless articles anyway. I don't think I'd ever seen anyone entertained by it for an entire flight, including one of this minimal duration.

The acceleration was phenomenal as we charged down the tarmac. I found it to be a huge rush of adrenalin, and could hardly imagine the exhilaration felt by an Air Force fighter pilot.

True to the Captain's word, the beverage carts were wheeled out on cue, one starting at the back of the plane and the other at the front. The lovely Mandy was beginning at the business class section, and George was taking it from the back; a position I was convinced he was more than partial to! As I was situated virtually in the middle of the plane, it was basically a coin toss as to whether Mandy or "Boy George" would be serving me a beverage. I wasn't a religious person, but found myself praying that the business class folks were content enough for now with their pre-flight drinks.

Like a slow puncture, my hope was being gradually deflated, as Mandy was giving the higher-paying passengers the utmost attention and quite rightly so. She looked like she was on good form, buttering up the male executives, giggling at appropriate intervals, flicking her bobbed style blonde locks from around her ears, and as a result, guaranteeing repeat business from these guys who were more than delighted by a fresh piece of female attention.

Our man George was making his way up the aisle at a rapid rate of knots; almost severing elbow joints on the way with his killer cart. He seemed completely unaware of the torture he was putting the unfortunate passengers through. It wasn't even neck and neck. He was at least eight rows ahead of Mandy in terms of progress. I carefully tucked my elbow to the inside of the armrest as he drew level with me.

"Can I interest you in a beverage?" he said to me with a smile and a slightly lingering stare. It was an add-on that only increased the near violation I'd experienced from his seatbelt inspection.

"I'll take a Heineken please."

"Coming right up," he said with yet another grin.

I watched as he cracked open the stumpy green and silver can, and topped up the small plastic glass that was more suitably sized for a shot of liquor than a cold beer. He carefully handed me the glass together with the can, which had more than half the content remaining.

"That'll be two pounds please."

I dug deep into my pockets for some change. I knew there was plenty in there as I'd removed a bunch of it and dumped it into one of the little grey plastic trays prior to going through the security scan.

George continued on his elbow bashing journey and I sipped on my cold(ish) beer. It wasn't his fault, but it pissed me off the way airlines now charged for food and drinks. Long gone were the days where you could get off the plane after a flight with a full belly and a heavy buzz going without having dropped a dime. If I was an airline CEO I would add five or ten pounds to the ticket costs and waive any food and drink fees; and in turn use it as a cunning advertising campaign against the competition. You'd still be paying for it, but it would be transparent, and the consumer perception would be they were getting something for nothing!

The two bozos next to me sipped merrily on their Cognacs; it was the only rest they gave their yapping mouths. They had progressed on from their financial jibber-jabber and were now blabbering on about how local political leaders should deploy more creative "out of the box" thinking as a modern approach for tackling inner city poverty of ethnic minority groups, and a way of combating increasing crime rates. These nuggets would've struggled with "in the box" thinking, but it didn't stop them from pitching *their* "creative" suggestions.

"They need to think long-term. Why not create a tax break for ethnic minority women who conceive with Caucasian males? Dilute skin colors over time as a way of breaking down the race walls. It could eventually lead to *real* equal opportunity, particularly in the workplace," said comb-over boy, sounding rather pleased with himself.

"Good point," replied bozo two.

It's not a good point; it's flawed with issues. He's an idiot, so please stop encouraging him. You're every bit as much of a donkey if you genuinely believe it's a good point.

They were driving me crazy. It was time for a nap.

I awoke to the voice of the captain on the intercom system telling the flight crew to prepare for landing. George was like a greyhound out the traps as he made a final seatbelt run. I fluffed up the crotch of my loose pants, just as a little treat for him. No harm in having someone on this planet—male *or* female—believe I was extremely well endowed.

Folks reluctantly moved their seats to an upright position; a motion I wished I had to replicate, as I'd fallen asleep with the chair fully erect and my neck was feeling the consequences. I still managed a giggle though. "Move your seats to an upright position." What other option did coach class passengers have? There were only two positions; fully upright or a little less upright. The six inches of possible recline could hardly qualify as not being upright! The way they called it out and valued any non-compliance as a serious safety breach was a joke in my book. Fair enough if we were all essentially lying down like all the lucky neck pain free buggers in first class.

We very slowly filtered off the plane. It was likely the same idiots during the boarding process that were again hindering us on the way off. A guy with a freakily large head three rows in front was almost bursting one of the snake sized veins on his temple such was the strain being applied to remove the larger than regulation bag from the overhead. I chuckled again. Maybe he was a motorcycle rider and he'd brought his helmet with him! He eventually got there, but would've had an easier time pulling on one of my roll-neck sweaters!

"Swindon please," I said to the cab driver.

"Owz it gowin' mate," said the fat cockney driver as we made our way to the highway.

"Not bad chief."

"Scottish I assume."

"You assume correctly."

"Rangers or Celtic?"

Rangers and Celtic were the two largest soccer clubs in Scotland; more famous for religious bigotry than fast-flowing entertaining football.

"Rangers."

"Ah, the boys in blue. Ah'm a blues man meself; Chelsea froo and froo."

"Chelsea is a good side. I just wish Rangers were as talented."

We exchanged football chat for most of the forty minute journey. His name was Dave; and for once was a cab driver who I enjoyed talking with. Most of them yapped on about general topics such as the weather and the price of gas; hardly stimulating. Dave even switched off the fare meter about ten minutes from my destination as he had "enjoyed my company". It was an extremely nice gesture. I was expensing the journey anyway, so I heavily padded his tip as a sign of my appreciation.

The hotel was nothing like I'd imagined. Any previous experience I had was of big name places like a Marriott or Hilton. This place was situated on the outskirts of town and only had six rooms. To me it resembled more of a family owned bed and breakfast found in the Highlands of Scotland, which suited me down to the ground. It was more of a large house, but majestic all the same. It was a solid looking red brick structure with that south of England thatched roof that only added character to its almost countryside location.

The owner, Ronald, greeted me like I was a long lost member of his family, and carried my bag for me as we headed up a flight of stairs to my room; an execution of customer service that could've made the lessons learned log of any hotel chain.

Ronald was a proud owner, you could just tell. The place was immaculate in every way, no stone left unturned. There were even a couple of chocolate candies neatly placed on the fluffy bed pillows.

He was a quirky sort of guy. Meeting him in the street and being asked to guess his occupation, nine times out of ten "Accountant" would've been the words from your mouth. He had neatly trimmed short brown hair in a side parting, smartly dressed in a pale blue shirt and black slacks, and a pair of thin silver rimmed glasses that matched his slim facial structure perfectly.

It had been a long day of travel. My head hurt, but dull in comparison to my pulsating knees. It was time for bed, but I had a big day of interviews in the morning, so a bit of last minute revision was in order before I lay my head beside the candies.

I slept like a log and didn't want to move after I opened my rejuvenated eyelids. The beige pillowcase had a fresh wet stain on it as a result of my comatozed drooling; a nightly event for me.

I painfully walked Frankenstein style to the warmth of the finely tiled shower. The heavy jet pounded on my shoulder blades, giving almost instant relief. I redirected the jet to my throbbing knees. I didn't hold out much hope of an immediate reprieve, but it was worth a shot.

As much as I was in pain though, there were more important matters at hand. I was well prepared for the interview and was surprisingly calm. I packed my overnight bag and headed downstairs for some breakfast before the taxi arrived to take me to the work facility.

Ronald happily greeted me as I reached the bottom of the stairs.

"How did you sleep?"

"Like a baby thanks."

"Did you hurt your back or something?"

He'd obviously saw me shuffling side step down the stairs. I was in pain and was never very confident with stairs at the best of times. I always had a paranoid notion that I was going to misplace a step and go tumbling down head first and bust up my fake hip as well as my other brittle joints. That's why I always descended in a very cautious fashion.

I arrived at the work facility. The cab driver was back to the usual uninteresting type of character, yapping on about the weather; completely opposite from Dave who brought me from the airport.

The place was huge, and continued to grow in stature as I painfully made my way towards the entrance revolving doors. I was *feeling* like crap, but I was definitely *looking* smart. The dark green single breasted suit, finely pressed light green shirt and maroon tie with the silver checks on it really made me appear business like. My black brogue shoes were gleaming so much I could almost see my pale and thin reflection in them.

"Hi there. Brandon Wilkinson here to see Shane Sparks," I announced to the rather butch looking female security guard at the reception desk.

"No problem sir. One moment and I'll give him a call. Is he expecting you?" she said in a soft and sexy voice; the last thing I was expecting to match with her manly physique.

"Yes, I have a nine o'clock interview with him."

"If you take a seat he should be with you in a few minutes."

I happily parked myself in one of the black leather couches. It was good to take a load off. They certainly spared no expense when it came to lobby furnishings.

I hated waiting and the stomach butterflies were kicking in, but at least taking my mind temporarily off my aching joints. I was well prepared, but the sheer anticipation of the interview process was causing the flutters.

"Brandon?"

"Hi there."

"Shane Sparkes," he said, extending his hand for the customary shake; his grip anything but intimidating.

"Very nice to meet you Shane."

"Likewise. How was your trip down?"

"Excellent. Very comfortable and all went smoothly."

"Great. Well if you want to just follow me I have a conference room set-up for us. The plan for the day is three interviews. The first with myself, then I'd like our technical specialist Anthony to have a chat with you, and then finally Liz from our Human Resources department would like to meet with you."

"Sounds good."

We made our way through the open plan office. It was as though everyone stopped working for the few seconds it took us to reach the conference room as they checked out the potential new colleague. Maybe they weren't looking at me, but my mind wondered what they were thinking. Were they talking about my limp and scrawny physique?

The conference room was nice, but not a patch on the leather clad reception area. It was smartly arranged with a large rectangular wooden table and matching brown high back cloth type chairs. It wasn't how I'd imagined, and the large double door entrance was all glass, enabling the entire office workforce to have visual access to the proceedings.

"Would you like a cup of coffee?"

"That would be great."

Shane summoned a girl to the room with a wave of his hand. She quickly appeared and he gave her the order for a pot of coffee and a plate of cookies. Her name was Stephanie and I assumed she was the department secretary. She was a reasonably attractive girl dressed all in black, including a pair of twelve holed Dr. Martin boots. She was very gothic looking as her eye make-up looked like it had been applied thickly with a black marker pen. She certainly made me feel smartly dressed and I knew they couldn't fault me on my attire if this was a sign of the current dress code from department members.

Shane and I chatted freely as we sipped on our hot coffees. He asked the general type of questions I'd been expecting and I felt as though I was sailing through. We even exchanged a few laughs which only added to the flow.

Before I knew it an hour had passed. There was a fine knock on the glass door and a giant of a man stood there briefly before popping his head inside.

"Should I come back in a few minutes?" said the man mountain.

"No, we're just wrapping up. Come on in. Brandon, this is Anthony. He is our technical expert. He's going to cover the more technological part of our requirements."

"Nice to meet you Anthony."

"Nice to meet you Brandon."

We shook hands, and unlike the earlier limp exchange with Shane, I was lucky to escape without a few broken bones in my hand. His hands were like shovels; the type that could've easily held a basketball in his palm with his knuckles facing the ceiling.

Anthony *appeared* to be like one of the boys. I'd watched him ogle Stephanie's butt as she'd been summoned to the office by Shane earlier, so I hoped there would be a familiar connection that could possibly see me through should I potentially choke on any of his technical questions.

As it turned out he was a bit of a hard ass; asking several questions I hadn't even dreamed of preparing for. Fortunately I was a smart cookie and basically blew him away with the detail of my responses. One thing I was was intellectual and experienced with manufacturing environments, so there wasn't much that could be thrown at me that I couldn't adequately handle.

"Do you have any questions for me Brandon?"

"Well Anthony, just one," I replied, preparing myself to take a chance on his character from what I'd seen from his earlier antics.

"Supposing I get this job, where is a decent bar in this town to meet some good looking women?"

It was definitely a gamble, but he just gave off the vibe that he was a bit of a ladies man. I had no proof behind the assumption, but my experience over the years with the boys at home had alarm bells ringing.

"Well Brandon, the place is full of them. There really are too many to mention. Supposing you do get the job, we'll have to sample a few in order for you to find that out for yourself."

The response was music to my ears, and solidified my initial gut feeling. Only time would tell if my gamble would pay off.

The next and final interview with the Human Resources lady went equally well. Her name was Liz, and initially unknown to myself she was actually from just outside Glasgow in Scotland, not too far from my upbringing. We chatted about work stuff for about ten minutes before talking about the homeland. I was sure it was still part of the interview process to see if my personality would fit in to the working environment.

All was peachy though and I left the plant feeling very good about myself as I headed back with the typically dull cab driver to the airport for the short trip back to Scotland. Hopefully George the air steward and his killer cart wouldn't be looking after us on the return flight.

A mere two days had passed since the interviews. I sat bored to tears at the desk of my current job when the phone rang.

"Mr. Wilkinson?"

"Yes, speaking," I replied.

"Hi Mr. Wilkinson it's David Stevenson from Diamond Recruitment."

"David, how are you? I thought I recognized the voice."

"Great news for you Brandon; you obviously kicked ass at the interview and they tell me they'll be sending out an official offer for you later this afternoon."

The clouds of my dull and boring day began to clear and a ray of sunshine filled my heart. I could hardly contain my excitement, but tried as best I could to remain cool.

"That's excellent news David; how much they offering?"

David disclosed the pay offer and I nearly fell off the back of my seat. It was *way* more than I was making now.

"You must've really knocked their socks off. It's a super offer, one that even surprised me, but they obviously wanted to put something on the table that was hard to refuse."

"I'm sure telling them that I had another two interviews with other companies didn't hurt that."

"Oh you do, I had no idea."

"No I don't, but I figured if they liked me they would want to move fast and have to put a good package on the table."

"Nice thinking. So would you like me to unofficially tell them you are happy with the conditions and will likely be accepting in the next few days."

"Absolutely; I'm really looking forward to the challenge. David many thanks for setting this up for me."

"You're very welcome Brandon. It's been a pleasure doing business with you. Good luck."

I could hardly keep the smile off my face and was looking forward to telling my current manager that I'd be leaving the company. We'd see how well the big melon headed creep would get on then. I *would* miss some of the folks there, but it was time to move on to a new challenge.

The hardest thing was going to be leaving my family behind, but it wasn't like I was moving overseas or anything. I could visit on weekends. It was only about a five hour drive or I could even jump on a flight if I found the drive was going to be too much for my body to take. It was about time I manned up and created a little more independence for myself. Take the reigns instead of riding feet up in the carriage. As long as I lived around my family I was only going to rely on their assistance and grow ever lazier. It was definitely time to step up to the plate and start fending for myself.

They said they were happy for me, but the forced smiles on their faces told me clearly that they were worried. They had every right to be concerned as I did not look healthy. You could've slotted me into my father's golf bag, stuck a head cover on me and called me Mr. Three Wood. I really had to fatten up a little, which was going to be one of the more challenging things in light of being away from my mum's homemade meals.

The day to my new beginning was approaching fast, and I was starting to get a little nervous as the reality of the entire situation was setting in. Could I actually cope on my own?

Stop being a big girl and keep it together. This is the test of character that you've needed for a long time.

The big day finally arrived. I had all my possessions loaded into my small two door car. The interior was jammed, mainly with clothes and a few essential kitchen utensils. The only passengers in the front seat were a stack of sandwiches in a Tupperware container that my mother had packed for me and a six pack of mini coke bottles. They would keep my appetite—or what I had of an appetite—at bay for the five hour car journey.

Both my parents were there to see me off. I dug deep to hold back the tears, but the realization of how much I was actually going to miss them hit me like a baseball bat. My Mum didn't dig as deep and the tears flowed down her cheeks and made quick work of distorting her black eyeliner. I hugged her tightly and didn't want to let go. My Dad was holding it together like the true man he was, but I could tell that like me, he was going to miss me being around, and was going to be worried for a while until he at least knew I was settling into my new life. We hugged as well and my initial thoughts of what was going on inside his head couldn't have been far off as he squeezed me python-like and told me to "take care of myself." It was at that point I had to get into the car and head south as quickly as possible.

My parents are still unaware of this to this day, but the first thirty minutes of my journey were a complete disaster. My feelings had been *so* bottled up that I just had to let go immediately after I left them that day. I sobbed like a school girl for that half hour, seemingly unable to stop. I even tried to put on some happy music on the radio, but it seemed that every channel change only locked onto a sad sounding song that only added to the stream flowing down my face. I almost had to pull over to the side of the road. My vision was like it was raining torrentially outside and my wipers were broken, even though neither was the case.

My health was as bad as ever, but the new job was working out well. My boss Shane *actually* listened to my concerns and supported my recommendations; unlike melon head before him.

It had been close to a month since my first day and I had settled in well not only to the role, but socially also, making several new friends who I'd already become very close to.

Anthony turned out to be just as I'd tagged him during the interview process. He had a brilliant mind and was fun to work and learn from, but outside the office environment he was an absolute scream. He certainly was the life of the party, could consume enough beer to floor a Rhino, and always had a story to tell that had the group cracking up in fits of laughter.

My four closest friends were Robbie, Stevie, John and Paul. I was on the look-out for a George and Ringo just to complete the set! They were a great bunch of lads, but the irony of it all as far as working in England now was that none of them were English. Robbie was Welsh and the other three guys were from Scotland. John was a Glasgow native like myself, but Paul and Stevie were from Edinburgh on the east coast. As a result we had many a moment bursting each other's chops about Scottish football teams—Edinburgh and Glasgow having some fine rivalries.

Like my mother had worried about, my eating habits left a lot to be desired. McDonalds were doing a roaring trade from my bank account, and although it wasn't exactly nutritional excellence, it was certainly better than not eating at all. I did have evenings though when the chronic pain was so much that I couldn't stomach anything, but I had learned that this was a cycle that was almost impossible to free myself from.

I continued to be a stubborn-headed pig though. The office parking lot was vast in size, and my time keeping in the morning wasn't exactly stellar as it took me an age to drag my stiff limbs out of bed and get into my clothes. As a result I was rarely able to get a parking spot anywhere near the main office entrance, meaning a walk of around three hundred yards before I was finally able to escape the usual rainy elements. Although that distance would never be considered anything more than a minute or less walk for most, it was anything but for me. There were days where I would have to pause for a brief break before being even halfway there. The pain at times was excruciating, every step feeling as though I was walking barefoot on a bed of nails as it sent sharp jolts through my entire lower half. I could've filled out the appropriate paperwork to have a disabled car tag and have the luxury of freely parking in the spots next to the front door, but for one, I viewed that as the lazy way out. I needed to push myself. I wanted to fight through the pain and hope that the walking would in turn help to loosen up the seized joints. Secondly I hated the perception of having everyone seeing me park in the handicapped zone. I didn't want the extra attention of folks wondering what was wrong. I already had eyes on me, but could palm it off with my usual knee injury story. I wanted to be normal and was paranoid enough without adding to it further. It was a dumb decision to make, but I couldn't let it go.

The company had paid for a small one bedroom apartment for me during my first month and that term was quickly coming to an end. I was thankful of that as it was anything but luxurious and not particularly user friendly to someone with my condition.

It was located at the end of a row in a cul-de-sac and it was a very peaceful setting, backing onto a small park set-up for kids. The most noise I'd hear in the evenings was from children playing merrily on the swings as their parents pushed them and they shouted "higher, higher." I recalled the days when that was me; happy as a pig in shit without a care in the world.

There was an upstairs to the apartment that I rarely used. The staircase was *extremely* steep and had a weird spiral affect as it neared the top floor, making it even more difficult than usual to navigate down. I was terrified of falling, particularly as there was nobody there to hear my cries should anything disastrous occur. As a result I slept on the downstairs sofa most nights. I was so stiff in the mornings, so the idea of tackling the abrupt and winding steps was something I avoided like the plague.

My usual evening routine was to take a bath upstairs (there was no luxury of a downstairs bathroom) and then make my way back down for the night. I would sit on the top step and slide myself down one stair at a time. It was a laborious process, but the safest approach given the circumstances.

I kept my toothbrush and other toiletries beside the kitchen sink, which was generally the most action that room ever saw. I was never much of a cook and generally would stop for take-out food on my way home from work rather than prepare any meal from scratch.

It was certainly rough living, but things could always be worse. I had to keep reminding myself of that. To any homeless person it would've been like spending life at the Ritz Carlton.

It was time to begin the search for a new place to live, preferably a single floor bungalow style or even a shared occupancy with a roommate; I could certainly use the company and somebody to be there to help me during troubling times.

Drink, Drugs and Tobacco

It felt almost like a weird strain of necrotizing fasciitis; a little evil inflammation bug munching heartily on my cartilage, eroding it away slowly, together with my already fragile state of mind. Why I thought alcohol was the answer still baffles me, but it strangely seemed to numb the pain where prescription drugs had failed.

I was now sharing a semi-detached rented house in the same town as the previous hideous apartment. It was about a ten minute drive from work and the same again to the center of town. The location was good, but the house was a little run down and needed some serious work. As we were only renting, that wasn't going to happen, the precise opposite in fact, as red wine spills, cigarette burns and fluid stains I didn't even want to ask my flat mate about, littered the washed out carpet and lint covered sofa. The exterior walls were very bland, a shitty looking brown-colored rough cast complimented elegantly with the torn guttering! The entire estate looked the same, rows and rows of these bleak cookie-cutter style terraced housing. They did match the weather well though and even seemed fitting with the dismal rainy winter days and matching wind chill welcomed only by penguins and polar bears.

I'd met my flat-mate Stevie at work and our personalities clicked immediately. We were both unattached, so figured sharing a place would be a good idea as it would save us a fortune on rent in the long run. He was a tall, well built, handsome looking fellow Scot, with well-defined chiseled features, and a heart of gold to match. He was a real manly man, loved his football, ladies—generally many of them—as well as beer, which he consumed in quantities that would've floored even the most seasoned of campaigners.

"Brandon, you up for a pint?"

"Yeah, no worries, nothing else going on," I said, flicking almost trance like through the endless TV channels of complete crap.

It was the truth—there was nothing else going on. I was single, work was done for the day, and it was either go out drinking or sit at home fighting the urge of feeling sorry for myself, and potentially cascading deeper into the cavern of depression.

The doctor's advice was to stay off alcohol while I was on my current medication; directions I decided against following. It wasn't the smartest decision of my life, but in my mind things couldn't get much worse. Going to the bar was the only real interaction I had with my current friends and I wasn't about to give that up as I had nothing else in my pathetic existence.

My buddies would play soccer after work, two nights per week, and although I would go along and sit on the sidelines, it wasn't the same. I'd watch in envy as they passed the ball around, eager to participate. In my day I would've controlled the field, as I took after my father as far as physical endurance and ball control. My spirits dropped as they missed chance after chance against the opposing team. I knew I would've buried almost every one of the opportunities had I been able to play.

My only outlet for contribution was joining them in the bar for the customary after match beers; something I *could* still contend at.

They were fairly heavy drinkers, visiting the bar almost every evening, and my fondness for Guinness was growing by the minute. The prospect of an evening in the pub was often the only thing that got me through the daily office grind.

My bad habits were on the increase as I took up smoking as well. Stevie, John, and Paul were all smokers, and would plough their way through a pack each on most evenings, and it wasn't long before I joined the trend. What was it going to do, kill me? Probably over time it would, but my thinking was now very short term, virtually day to day, so I didn't care. My thoughts of ending my life were all but gone, but I didn't particularly want to live into my seventies or eighties, crippled with the disease, wheelchair bound, regularly pissing my pants, and counting on others to help me through each day. No, I would ride it out for as long as I could, but should my years end prematurely due to alcohol or smoking-related illness, then so be it.

The guys truly were great friends and always will be. John was a wonderful and caring man, who was always up front with his feelings, and made it perfectly clear that he was there for me whenever I needed him. He was a typical West End of Glasgow character; no beating around the bush, and would've fought Goliath for you should the situation arise. He was doing well for himself at work; a short stocky guy, dark hair, with sharp features, and well known for getting the job done in the office and making things happen; a true Scottish terrier.

Paul was also an extremely close friend, and the first guy I'd really hung out with since moving to England. He was a typically pasty-looking guy from the East coast of Scotland. He was tall and slim with dark brown hair in a similar style to the Gallagher brothers from the band Oasis. His skin was pale enough that it appeared as though it would take two weeks sunbathing in the Bahamas to get it up to white. I had a lot of respect for Paul and admired the way he treated me. He knew I was in constant pain, but was more of the type to push me along rather then give me the sympathy card. He was tough, but deep down I knew he cared, and that meant a lot to me.

Our lifestyles were as unhealthy as they could possibly be, and would never be detailed in a Men's Health article unless is was a story on what not to do. With the exception of John, we were all single guys, far from home, and the Scottish culture in general revolves around drinking, so it was essentially a given that we would conduct ourselves in the path we were following.

I was never really one for doing drugs, but one evening Stevie got hold of some cannabis, and produced the large clear plastic bag of "gear" as we were sipping on a few beers at home, prior to making our way out to the bar. He sat in his usual slouched position in the stained brown armchair next to the TV and gave the three of us a master class on how to roll a joint. It wasn't like anything I'd seen before; not your typical thin two skinner, this was more like a big fat work of art, and would've been at home on the set of Dances with Wolves; Kevin Costner looking on well impressed as "Ten Bears" passed this humungous peace pipe to one of his fellow tribe.

Stevie took a few extended inhales and passed to me.

"Get some of that in you," he said in a high pitched voice, before exhaling a massive cloud of smoke.

"Not for me chief," I said, extending the roll-up towards an eagerly awaiting Paul.

"It's good for the old arthritis. I saw a program about it on TV the other night," replied Stevie.

This intrigued me, so I pulled back my hand from Paul's direction; the joint still firmly between my middle and index fingers.

"I'm listening."

"I don't know exactly what it does, but a bunch of folks like yourself were raving about it. They said it worked better than any pain reliever they got over the counter; probably worth a try. It'll give you a good buzz as well, so sounds like a win win situation if you ask me."

Without further hesitation I took an almighty drag, and in hind sight, probably a little too much for a first attempt, as I felt it burn the back of my throat, which was swiftly followed by a fit of coughing that could've passed as the antics of someone who'd been smoking two packs a day for the last fifty years.

The boys erupted with laughter, as did I, but this was short-lived as I felt an almost instantaneous rush to my head that nearly caused me to pass out. My brain felt so light as I sank back on the couch and the tingle quickly swept across my entire body like a fast acting disease.

"Holy shit," I said, finally passing the roach over to Paul.

"Some good gear isn't it," said Stevie with a smile.

"I'll say; I can feel it hitting me already. It's good though. It's almost like I could just float away,"

The plump cigarette took another three laps around our little four man circle.

"I'm absolutely mashed," said John. He paused for a second before erupting into laughter.

It was infectious, as all of us followed suit. The more we laughed, the harder it was to stop. Nothing funny had actually happened, but it was like something had crawled inside us and flicked on the giggle switch.

"Ready for a few pints then?"

"Paul, as long as I can get my limp body out of this chair."

Again we laughed uncontrollably at what wasn't even a joke.

We locked the door and stumbled down the street towards the Crown bar at the end of the road.

I was very thoughtful as we walked, vision slightly impaired, but there was a relaxed feel about me that was hard not to enjoy. Why was cannabis illegal anyway? If it really had magical pain relieving properties, why shouldn't we use it to our benefit? I was feeling so calm and at peace with the world. To me alcohol was a far more dangerous addiction, and had also been the root cause for many violent exchanges I'd encountered in bars over the years. I knew of many guys who were like Jekyll and Hyde. The finest and friendliest folks when they were sober, but as soon as they were drunk it seemed to trigger a violent streak within them; it was baffling. Right now I was *so* mellow, and the last thing on my mind would've been to inflict any pain on anyone. Hugging them to death was certainly an option, but I hadn't read too many newspaper articles with the headline "Man asphyxiates fellow colleague after cannabis smoking binge". I had to agree with Stevie; it did seem like a win win on many fronts.

It became like a nightly ritual; home from work, smoke a joint, wolf down a can of soup and two slices of toasted cheese, then head down the street with Stevie and Paul for a few beers and half a pack of cigarettes. John would join us a couple of times a week, but married life for him wasn't an obstacle we had to endure.

It was a rough lifestyle, and not one I'd recommend, but any negatives on my internal organs were outweighed by the positive effects on my ailing joints. The one good thing on my side was the monthly blood check that was a routine requirement for my condition. They checked inflammation levels as well as a bunch of other components I had no knowledge of, but it was nice to know they were keeping tabs on me. The one element they assessed that I *was* appreciative of was the liver function test. The fact they were regularly looking at this removed any guilt or concern about the alcohol consumption while taking my medication. Drinking can affect the liver, but if there were any issues, they would likely be picked up on quickly and I could put a stop to it before it was too late.

Right now though, anything that could help me was a winner, legal or otherwise. Deep down I didn't want to be a marijuana smoker, but it was working for me where pharmaceuticals were failing.

Days were painful and long. I never smoked it before work in the morning, even as much as I was tempted or indeed wanted. I couldn't risk being disciplined or fired for being stoned. I didn't think they would've been receptive to the reasoning that I was almost pain free as a result and in turn significantly more productive.

Every day was a struggle, and by five o'clock in the evening I couldn't get a joint in my hand quickly enough. By that time I was in acute pain and the pot was way more effective for me, and more importantly, fast-acting, than a couple of anti-inflammatory pills.

I pushed for new treatment at every doctor's visit. Surely there was something more effective that could cause me to drop the marijuana smoking?

Finally they prescribed me a one week dose of steroid pills. I'd walked in to the rheumatologist's office like a frail old man; pale, skinny, bent over and hobbling along in miniature steps. My knees were swollen like a couple of baseballs and felt like they were burning inside; the inflammatory liquid bubbling away like molten lava.

The look on the staff's faces was priceless. I could tell they were a little disturbed to see a young man in such a state. It was a little sad that such extreme physical incapability had to be the trigger point for a different course of action.

It was like a miracle. The day after popping four of the Prednisone I felt as good as new. The swelling had subsided and it was as though they'd also had a strange lubricating effect on my joints, as my range of motion had increased exponentially. This may have only been a temporary reprieve, but I was determined to make the most of it.

The boys were a little surprised by the announcement that I'd be joining them in town for the evening at "The Barn" nightclub. I typically avoided those establishments like the plague. I wasn't able to dance due to the arthritis, and the packed crowds were a deterrent on their own, as there were only enough seats for about one in ten, and I generally could only put up with standing for fifteen minutes max. Not tonight though; I was ready for action.

The line to get into The Barn was typically long, but Stevie was well acquainted with the doorman who resembled a white version of Mike Tyson; fully equipped with the biceps, no evidence of a neck, and the girly sounding voice to match. He was the dealer who sold Stevie his dope, and was responsible for much of my pain relief. As a result, we skipped the queue and were swiftly ushered inside, much to the resentment of the complaining masses.

The place was banging. The DJ was positioned high up in his enclosed podium above the packed dance floor, spinning and mixing his techno tunes like a conductor to his enthusiastic orchestra below as they rhythmically moved in time to every beat he created.

We patiently pushed our way to the bar and Stevie ordered a tequila shot and beer for me, John, Paul and himself. We toasted my surprising presence and threw the fire water back, followed by the obligatory facial spasm and body shiver that resembled some of the ongoing dance floor moves, before heading to a quieter spot with our beers in order to check out some ladies.

The talent was magnificent. There was no doubt the combination of dull lighting and carefully applied make-up was enhancing the beauty scores, but perhaps the lighting was boosting *our* attractiveness as well.

Although I was feeling a lot better, I was still very self-conscious with my appearance. The darkness may have been effective as far as disguising a few pimples or even some wonky teeth, but for me it wasn't going to help add thirty wanted pounds. I just had to hope someone had a fetish for short, skinny, and gaunt-looking guys. I decided if that one came off I was definitely buying a lottery ticket!

We took our position close to the top of the staircase that led up from the dance floor. It was a superb vantage point as many lovely girls filtered back and forth.

I'd picked a bad night to wear a black shirt, as the purple fluorescent light emphasized a bunch of white speckles on the chest and shoulders, making it appear as an extreme dandruff problem that only added to my self-consciousness.

As usual, Stevie was in fine form. He and Paul were like an Abbott and Costello double act, and John wasn't exactly a member of the shy department when it came to flirting.

A cute blonde with a perfect bobbed haircut almost tripped on her face as she got to the top of the stairs. The six inch clear high heels combined with the alcohol over indulgence being the obvious root cause.

"I knew you were going to fall for me, but I didn't expect it to be this early in the night," said Stevie with a smile as he grabbed her hand, making sure she was steady on her feet.

"Thanks honey," she replied, staring deep into his welcoming eyes.

She was definitely cute, but disproportionate looking—in a good way. Her deep red glossy lipstick combined with the sculpted blonde hair was divine, but she was no more than five feet tall and ninety pounds, twenty of which appeared to be located in her bra!

"Honey? So somebody's told you how good I taste?"

The line was a little cheesy to say the least, but she was lapping it up like a weary desert nomad quenching himself at an overdue oasis.

"No they didn't, but maybe I should find that out for myself."

"I agree. Let's step in to my office."

Unbelievable. Off they went together, hand in hand towards the bar. He turned as he led her on their way and fired a wink and a smirk followed by a quick raise of the eyebrows. We stood there open-mouthed, exact replicas of the two friends she'd left behind.

"If only I found it that easy," said Paul, directing his comment towards the little blonde's friends.

"Well, you never know until you try," replied the taller of the girls.

"You dancing?" said Paul with a twinkle in his eye.

"You asking?"

"I'm asking."

"I'm dancing."

Off they went down the stairs, just as the DJ chilled the tunes down to more of a house vibe.

They looked a nice match, both tall and slim, and not dissimilar either with their Oasis haircuts. She did suit it though; a look not all women could pull off.

I was determined not to be outdone, so decided to take an extremely direct approach with the remaining girl who was left standing there like a long lost soul.

"Come on, let's go," I said to chick three, taking her hand and leading to the stairs.

Much to my delight, her hand remained limp and offered no resistance. I wasn't sure if my messed up mind could've dealt with any rejection.

"I'll be here on my own when you guys are done," shouted John sarcastically as we made our way carefully down the stairs. I didn't feel bad for him and I knew he didn't care. His lovely wife Elaine was at home with the kids and he was very much in love with her, and wouldn't have even dreamed of dancing with another girl never mind anything else. His beer was almost full anyway, so it gave him some time to catch up with the rest of us.

I was surprised how easy I sailed my way down the stairs. The Prednisone pills really were something. If anything, the girl on my arm, Tina, was in fact slowing me down. It was like a balancing act as she meticulously placed each huge plat-form shoe down on the floor. You would've thought she was tiptoeing her way through a mine field.

Tina would've never taken first prize at the beauty pageant, but seeing as I was no oil painting myself, conditions were perfect. Fortunately for me she was short, about a couple of inches less than me, and that was including the Spice Girls shoes she was sporting—which seemed to be a running theme within this group of chicks. I was a stickler for not being watched with a woman taller than me, and with my paranoia already on overdrive, was another variable I was glad I didn't need to contend with.

Tina had one thing going for her in her pearly white smile. She was a little bottom heavy and flat-chested, but her smooth pretty face made up for any short-fall in the physique department.

My dancing was awful—a mixture of my father's rhythm and the free flowing movement of the Tin Man from Wizard of Oz. Fortunately the floor was packed and assisted perfectly in disguising my obvious lack of talent. There wasn't room to swing a cat, so I just moved my feet in baby steps to the beat and smiled occasionally in Tina's direction.

"THIS IS CRAZY DOWN HERE. YOU WANNA GRAB A DRINK AT THE BAR?" I shouted to Tina. We were right next to the speaker system and the base was thumping, making it impossible to communicate unless you virtually had your tongue in the other person's ear!

"YEAH, IT'S A LITTLE TOO MANIC DOWN HERE."

We made our way back up to the awaiting John; Tina continuing the balancing act with her stilts footwear, although she was finding the upward climb a lot easier than the earlier descent.

John wasn't where we'd left him, but after a quick glance towards the bar we saw that all of the gang had already made their way over there. Stevie and little blondie were stuck to each other's faces like a couple of plungers. There was nothing slow and passionate about it, more like a dog fight.

Veronica, Stevie's tonsil hockey opponent surfaced for air and had a quick confab with her buddies before excusing themselves to the bathroom; no doubt for a status report on us guys as much as to drain off some of the alcohol.

The group trip to the toilet was one thing guys would never replicate. I could just imagine the look on Paul and John's face if I asked them if they fancied joining me for a pee!

"Right lads, I think it's time we drank up and went somewhere else," said Stevie with a look of resignation on his face.

"Are you nuts? You're *totally* in there," replied John rather confused.

Paul and myself were similarly perplexed.

"I'm in there alright, just as long as I'm happy with a night of making out. Don't get me wrong, she's got a tongue like an electric eel, but she's made it very clear she doesn't believe in sex before marriage. So drink up and let's go before they get back; unless you two boys are having any more success?"

"Not me. She seems more concerned about breaking a nail or having some hair out of place than giving me any attention," said Paul.

It was all on me.

"Let's go. I wasn't too mad about mine anyway, and I think the feeling was mutual. I was just happy to have *any* form of female interaction tonight, and my thirst has been quenched. Let' go to The Crown for a few," I replied, hoping they would go for my suggestion. I was in my comfort zone there.

"Done! Right, let's get the hell outta here," signaled Stevie pointing to the exit, swigging down the remainder of his beer, one eye fixed on the ladies bathroom door.

It turned out to be a good night. I was happy we ended up back at our local bar. It was more my scene and we didn't have to scream across the room in order to be heard.

We sat at our usual table in the corner and chatted about everything and nothing. My mood was extremely upbeat, and to be able to sit around pain free was a rare treasure. My only wonder was how long it would continue.

Over a week passed and the steroid pills had been finished a few days back, but so far so good. Life was fun again, and I'd even substituted the marijuana smoking for walking around the neighborhood; it was a much healthier form of recreation. I didn't do anything too strenuous, but walked long enough to cover the time it would've taken to polish off two shared joints. I'd breathe in the fresh air as I walked. I'd forgotten how invigorating it was. Even breathing in the odd funky smell as I passed some garbage cans wasn't all that bad; I was free again and savoring every moment.

I awoke, sunlight beaming through the blinds in horizontal stripes; one catching me directly in the face as I prized open my crusty eyelids. It was another lovely day, or at least it was until I attempted to clamber out of bed.

A cloud must've covered the sun and sent the room into a moment of darkness. It mirrored my mood as my heart raced, spirits crashed, and the familiar acute pain was once again back with me.

Damn you arthritis. A one week vacation! Thanks very much you bastard. You could've at least had the decency to take a month holiday. I'm sick of the sight of you. There was so much I still wanted to do.

I openly wept. The last ten days had been like old times again, but I was now back to struggling to even make it out of bed. I knew these tears had been coming. I knew the steroid pills were only going to be a temporary Band-aid on this incurable wound, but it still hurt; like extra salt being rubbed in.

Somebody please help me.

Chronic Pain—In the Ass

Most folks encounter physical pain in their lives, whether it's a bad headache, stomach cramps or even a serious sports injury. But many are unaware of the effects of living with chronic pain, which affects fellow arthritis sufferers, cancer victims, as well as many other conditions. Most people's general pain goes away, or is sporadic enough not to result in a complete mental character makeover.

I was like Jekyll and Hyde at times. There were many days I'd experience a complete cocktail of emotions; everything from anger, depression, anxiety, withdrawing myself from social interaction, as well as general crankiness, which was likely a result of the overpowering fatigue I was fighting.

The severe pain and stiffness caused varying sleep patterns. Most nights were spent painfully tossing and turning, attempting to find a position that could be tolerated for the evening. Even on the nights where I felt I'd had a wonderful sleep, I would wake up completely exhausted.

I had always been one for dreaming, but the activity levels they now contained were almost off the charts. In this fantasy world I was free to run, jump and generally take my physical abilities to where they'd been before my diagnosis. I was back playing football again, sinking a barrel load of birdie putts and competing again in martial arts at the highest level of competition.

I had to research this phenomenon as I was totally perplexed by it all. The results were fascinating to me. The dreams were *so* lifelike, feeling as though I had actually lived the events again. Medical journals said that there are times when the body responds to dreams in this way, which can in turn lead to an exhausted feeling in the morning as well. It was like a Catch 22 situation. Lack of sleep led to fatigue, but when I actually got a good night's rest I was going through the motions like I was a kid again, which resulted in exhaustion when I woke up also!

This was another reason for alcohol. I either couldn't sleep or when I did I awoke equally as tired. The drinking at least removed the former, which was the worst of the two options. Being unable to sleep just caused more pain as I moved uncomfortably around and would have an array of negative thoughts that only enhanced the depression and anxiety. At least when I was drunk I just passed out almost coma like until the morning. I was still tired when I woke up, but at least it prevented the unwanted thoughts and scenarios that flooded my mind.

The fatigue though was the least of my worries. The mood swings were the worst. As I got down on myself I often became angry, snapping at colleagues and family members completely out of the blue. It wasn't their fault, I was just bitter. It was back to the old question of "why me?" and being unable to carry out the most menial of tasks that had previously been taken for granted. This in turn added to my depression; mad at myself for snapping at those who actually cared for me and hating the person I was becoming at times.

Emotional distress can make pain worse and it was killing me. There seemed like no way out. Work was getting the better of me as I was often late as a result of taking an eternity to get out of bed in the morning, and when I was there, found it hard to stay focused on the daily activities—they seemed so trivial to me in the overall scheme of things. This in turn didn't assist with the pain management. Regardless of this I made it to the office everyday. I was determined to fight.

Don't let it beat you Brandon, you're tougher than that. Screw them all. Don't worry what they are thinking about you. The people who really care are behind you in this battle.

A warm bath always helped, although it occasionally took as long to get in and out of the tub than it did getting out of bed in the morning. The warm water and silky bubbles temporarily relieved my troubles though, and when I eventually managed to clamber into the water, the physical obstacle course of getting there in the first place seemed all worthwhile. I could almost feel the heat submitting the inflammation into defeat as I lay there soaking; often sparking up a pre-prepared cannabis joint as I did so. The mellowing effect of this combination was like heaven to me, and I was worry free in the solitude of my own little steam and smoke filled room. Life was good at these times, and even when the water began to cool, I would empty some out and refill with some piping hot goodness.

Lightweight

My weight was becoming a serious issue. For a while I was aware I was losing some, but it was spiraling out of control. I couldn't eat. The pain made me feel sick to the stomach and all I could deal with at times was Cup a Soup; not exactly the most nutritious of snacks. The only times I ate like a pig was after I was stoned. That gave me an attack of the munchies, but was generally satisfied with a family sized bag of Cheetos and four chocolate chip cookies, hardly a well balanced meal either. I needed to be eating steak and eggs for breakfast, a tuna salad for lunch and a hearty dinner, but that sensible ideal never came to fruition. The only part of me showing a bit of weight gain was my stomach; in light of the six pints of Guinness I would put back on a nightly basis, completely against doctor's orders.

I was on a medication by the name of Methotrexate. I was moved onto this drug in combination with an anti-inflammatory called Naproxen. The previous medication—Sulfasalazine—had been a complete failure, and Methotrexate was the next in line for trial. I was warned at the time not to take alcohol while I was on this as there was possibility of an interaction. Methotrexate had the potential side affect of damaging the liver, and alcohol is renowned all over the globe for having a similar ability. I didn't care though. What else did I have? In my mind my life was over, and the regular liver checks gave me a false sense of security.

What I needed to do was eat. I was 150 lbs prior to diagnosis and I was down to around 120 lbs right now. I saw myself in the mirror every morning and wasn't aware of the significance of the physical changes I was *really* going through. I knew the weight was dropping, but to me I didn't know how drastic it was until a visit back home to Scotland one weekend.

The drive home was a long one, maybe not in the minds of most, but five or six hours sitting in essentially the same position was like a death sentence to me. The stiffening effect on my joints was incredible. Even the short ten minute drive to work in the morning had a similar impact to waking up in the morning—stiff as a poker and the complete loss of will to continue breathing.

The journey, although long, was a straight forward one. Highway all the way, which was good in many ways, but led to extreme boredom. Although I was in pain, the closer I got to home, the more I became motivated. I missed my family dearly and knew they were waiting eagerly to see me and I'd be taken care of like a King for the weekend. My mouth watered at the prospect of some of my Mother's homemade soup—I *was* hungry and it was one of the few things I was able to stomach.

About twenty minutes from home I called them.

"Hey Dad, it's me."

"Hey son, where are you?"

"Just passing Lanark right now, I should be there in about fifteen to twenty minutes."

"How you feeling?"

"Pretty good. Getting a bit stiff though."

I was such a liar. There was nothing pretty good about it, but I'd made a deal with myself to remain positive in their eyes. I was down enough for ten people but wanted them to feel that I was making some progress—at least mentally.

"Well it won't be long now."

"I know. Just tell Mum to get the soup on," I said with a forced laugh.

"It's ready and waiting for you son."

"Great, can't wait. I'll talk to you shortly."

"Take it easy."

"Will do Dad."

He had a warmth in his voice that told me he was missing me and was really looking forward to seeing me. I was *so* lucky to have them both. I pressed on the accelerator, pushing it up to 85 mph. I wanted to get home as quickly as I could and didn't give a crap if I was pulled over for speeding. To me a ticket was just a trivial matter in light of everything else in life.

I cried as I passed the other drivers on the road. I loved my family. I hated myself for causing them daily worry, but was blessed to have two parents who would've died for me if it meant I could be pain free.

Growing up I went to a high school with a very strange mix of students. Most were from working class backgrounds, a few were from very well-to-do families and many were from the part of town renowned for its high crime and unemployment rates. My family was middle of the road. They had worked hard for everything they'd achieved, and due to my Mum's financial astuteness, had reached a point in their lives where they were fairly comfortable. This was not the case for many of the kids from the poverty stricken area of town. Who knew what they were doing right now. I'd heard that a few of them were in jail for burglary and drug related crimes, one was dead as a result of an overdose, and another had lost his mind completely and was now living in a padded room in one of the surrounding mental institutions. I was *so* thankful I didn't grow up in such an environment. Their parents didn't appear concerned with what they did growing up. I may have been suffering, but at least I had a loving family. A feeling of being alone and uncared for in the world would've been worse in my mind than any physical misfortune I was enduring.

My Dad was waiting outside for me in the parking lot of their apartment building as I pulled into a vacant spot. His previous upbeat tone was replaced with a look of initial shock as he set eyes on me.

It had been several weeks since I'd last seen them, and the weight loss during that time must've been far more striking to him than it had been to me.

"Oh, son," he said, helping my stiff skeleton out of the driver seat and giving me a huge hug. He gripped me so tightly it hurt, but I bit my upper lip and held in the pain.

"I know I've lost a few pounds, but I think it's this new medication. My appetite sucks, but I'm feeling not too bad," I said, struggling to keep my emotions in check, and a little guilty about lying regarding the medication. My appetite had already gone prior to the medication switch, but I didn't want to admit that it was pain related as I'd been telling them things were a lot better—not daring to reference the marijuana of course!

He grabbed my weekend bag and I put my arm around his shoulder as we made our way up the stairs to their front door. I palmed off my current pain and stiffness to the effects of the car journey, and although he found it plausible, I could tell he was figuring out I wasn't being *completely* truthful with them.

My mother's reaction was also one of shock.

Maybe you really are looking even sicker.

"That's it, you are going to eat well while you are here this weekend," she said as her eyes filled up with tears.

"Well I will if you're doing the cooking," I joked. I always had the defense mechanism of following up with some humor to deflect from the concern.

"Oh I'll make sure you eat. Go and take a seat on the couch and I'll bring in some soup," she replied, also giving me a tight hug and a big kiss on the cheek.

I was exhausted as I sank into their soft white leather couch with one of the matching cushions propped behind my painful back.

Back pain was becoming a major issue also. It wasn't *really* joint related, but it was definitely a byproduct of my poor posture, which *was* joint related. My busted knees and resulting limp had my center thrown off completely, and even the shortest of walks around the high street or a venture up the corridor to the work cafeteria had my lower spine screaming at me to take a rest.

"Well it doesn't look like this new medication is doing you much good either," said my mum as she brought in the soup on my favorite tray, which was also stacked with six slices of buttered bread. She really was going to try everything to put a few pounds on me.

"I know, but I've been doing not too bad other than the weight."

"Well it's not good enough. You look terrible Brandon. I hate seeing you like this, it really breaks my heart. I'm going to start looking into other alternatives. I don't want to see you suffering anymore."

The tears began trickling down her face.

Sandy the Faith Healer

Desperate times require desperate measures, and these were desperate times. I had lost all faith that had ever existed in my life, but ironically enough I'd reluctantly agreed to visit a faith healer. What was there to lose? We'd tried everything else to enable a better, more manageable existence, and I could see the thread of hope in my mother's eyes as she told me of the success stories achieved from Sandy's magical hands.

Sandy was a friend of the family, and a member of the Musselburgh bowling club that my Aunt Eleanor was also involved with. They were very competitive, but it was more of a social thing, backed up by the after match drinking in the clubhouse which was more than encouraged by the working class prices.

Eleanor set up the appointment and my mother accompanied me on the first visit. The thirty mile drive to Musselburgh, Edinburgh was a quiet and anxious affair—I was actually a little nervous and locked in a daydream for most of the journey, missing out on some of the beautiful scenery along the way. I had no idea what to expect, but had visions of Sandy with a long grey beard, almost wizard-like in appearance, ready to deliver serious volumes of stress relieving "hocus pocus" to my ailing joints.

"We're here," said my mother, awakening me from my trance, sounding a little surprised as she assessed the surrounding neighborhood.

"Are you sure?" I said, equally as baffled.

"I'm pretty sure. It matches the address and directions Eleanor gave me."

We tentatively headed to the brown front door with matching exterior "Welcome" mat. It was the end house on a council terraced row; a very dull and bleak setting seemingly void of wizardry or any other healing qualities to say the least. There was an eerie quality as we neared the door though, that temporarily restored my potential hope.

"Sandy?" I quizzically asked the small gentleman who answered the door.

"The very one; you must be Brandon, come on in."

"This is my mum, Betty."

"Hi Betty."

"Nice to meet you Sandy."

We all exchanged a handshake and made our way up the gloomy hallway. Sandy looked like he should be mending pipes or plastering walls, not displaying magical healing powers. He was about my height, short thinning brown hair, with a moustache speckled with the occasional silver looking strand. His place had a very homely feel to it, plain but cozy, with the smell of the evening's beef stew still very evident.

He ushered us through to the kitchen area, which on initial inspection reminded me of my grandmother's place. Similar with its fading, washed out yellow walls, nicotine tainted white ceiling, and old style electrical appliances; remnants of stew remaining on the spiraling heating element of the right hand ring of the stove top.

Situated in the corner was a brown leather massage style table, worn in a few places, and had obviously catered for many before me.

"I bet this table's seen a bit of action," I said, immediately wishing I could've taken back the words, as they hadn't quite come out how I'd intended. I was uncomfortable as it was, and hoped he didn't take it as an implication of sexual activity between his wife and himself. Even if it had been partial to a few games of "how's your father" with his lady, he continued on unfazed, much to my relief.

"I've treated half the bowling club on this table. Most of them are fifty and over, and partial to a few aches and pains. In fact it was here on this very table that I straightened out your Aunt Eleanor's neck trouble in about fifteen minutes. She hasn't had a single bit of bother since then, and it's done wonders for her bowling game. I wish I'd waited one more week before treating her though. Two days after I healed her she whipped my arse in the quarter finals of the club championship," he chuckled, but with a glint in his eye that screamed he was only partially joking.

It was Eleanor's success story that was the icing on the cake as far as convincing my family that Sandy was worth a shot. I could tell my dad was a little apprehensive, but Eleanor *was* a straight up person, a no bullshit type of character who never suffered fools gladly.

She'd been having an awful time with her neck, deteriorating her performance in the sport she loved, but was now back to her winning ways, holding her own and more against the men in the club. I was sure Sandy wasn't the only man cursing her recovery back to full fitness.

"So what's causing you the most problems?" inquired Sandy in a manner that mirrored every physician I'd ever visited.

"My knees are the worst. Every step I take makes me flinch, and I can't even fully straighten my legs anymore. It's causing me to lose all my thigh muscles as I'm not using them properly."

I wasn't joking either. I could've now doubled as a chicken with my slight, stalk-like limbs. If only I could've run around like one I would've been fine with them in their current condition. In my present state though, I wouldn't have placed in the 100 meters of the geriatric Olympics, even if half the participants were using zimmer frames.

"Pop off your jeans and hop up onto the table face up."

He was being optimistic to say the least. A firecracker wedged in my ass cheeks was the only way there would be any hopping onto tables. I removed my jeans in what appeared to be slow motion, every movement resulting in a sharp, needle-like pain attacking my body—I was struggling.

"I can do it!" I snappily said to my mum, as I saw her motioning to assist in the process. I hated myself for the way I spoke to her at times, as she only ever had my best interest at heart. I was fine with any aid when it was just us, but there was an embarrassment factor when others were present that seemed to automatically trigger an objection on my part. My mind was messed up, but I *could* do it—it just took time. It was excruciating, but I had to fight it and not lie down in submission.

I lay on my back after what seemed like an eternity since Sandy's original request. Although I was motionless, the pain was flowing through me like electricity. Gravity was not my friend, as it pushed down on my knees, attempting to straighten them, but my mind was resisting, and winning the battle for that matter. Sandy could see the pain from my furrowed brow, and kindly placed a thick, rolled up white bath towel under my knees for support, much to the relief of my pain sensors and strained wrinkled features.

"Relax your mind. Find a happy place, somewhere that brings joy to you."

I was surprised by this soothing, almost spiritual statement from a man on appearance who looked as tough as nails and blue collar by nature.

I quickly found my happy place, half surprising myself with where I ended up. It was with my dad, my friend. It wasn't a recent memory either, but one of the earliest bonding moments I could ever remember. I was six years old again, no worries in the world, and not even aware that a condition by the name of arthritis even existed. We were together on the golf course at a little seaside town called Montrose on the North East coast of Scotland—a true links. It was just after Tom Watson had won the Open Championship at Muirfield in 1980. I distinctly remember looking at the winning photograph in the Daily Record newspaper, Tom holding the famous Claret Jug aloft and his wife Linda planting a well earned kiss on his warm, cheerful looking face. I had no idea then, but staring back at this I realized it was then I was attracted to women. Her shiny black hair, and the fact she was kissing a boy caused some stirring from within me that was alien and unexplainable back then.

That day was a wonderful one as I swung from my mobile hips, cracking the ball down the tightly mown fairways using my cut-down, wooden shafted clubs that my father had prepared for such a day. On that occasion I was void of any swing thoughts; a skill that hackers today would pay good money for. I breezed my way around, hitting the ball for what I believed was miles, but probably no more than one hundred yards with my hickory shafted driver. One hundred and twenty one was my score for eighteen holes, meaningless to me at that time, but a score that would still be more than acceptable by around five percent of adult golfers today.

Sandy must've been working on me for at least ten minutes before I surfaced from my childhood recollection. He was applying a hot oil rub to my knees. It had began as a cold sensation, but quickly accelerated to a piping hot temperature. The relief was extremely pleasing and helped me to relax even further. Next he rubbed his hands together at an alarming rate and proceeded to move them ever so slowly over the top of my knees without actually touching them. At first I was a little confused by this, and even gave my mother a quick look, mentally sending the words "what the hell is this" in her direction. She raised her brows back at me, but almost instantaneously I was baffled by what occurred. There were a series of short, sharp, electric type shocks hitting my knee caps.

"Wow, what was that?" I said, looking at Sandy with a complete look of disbelief on my face.

"That's all part of the treatment I provide. Don't worry, your reaction is the same as everyone who sees me for the first time. I don't actually know how I do it either, but it is a gift I think I've been given for a reason. These are the pulses I generate that seem to have a healing affect on people."

"I have to admit Sandy, I was a little skeptical about coming here today, but that right there is enough to make me think otherwise."

I was truly impressed and it was like nothing I'd ever felt before. He wasn't even laying a finger on me, which was the most astonishing thing. Maybe this guy did have healing powers. I was never really a believer in spiritual healing, or anything for that matter that didn't actually involve pharmaceutical drugs, but my belief was being challenged right now and I was beginning to change my opinion with every miniature shock being delivered to my damaged joints.

He continued on for another twenty minutes or so before telling me that my time was up.

"That's enough for today. I actually cannot go on any longer. It's not that I don't want to, but giving this treatment saps the energy from me."

"Amazing Sandy, I'm still a little overwhelmed by all of this."

"You believe over time. Come back and see me the same time next week. It can sometimes take a few sessions before the treatment takes full effect."

I slowly but steadily sat up on the table and swung my legs over the edge before sliding myself onto my feet. There was no pain anymore; it was remarkable.

"Holy crap, I don't feel any pain right now."

It was unbelievable. I was in severe discomfort when I'd arrived, but now it had completely vanished.

"I can believe that. I'm just happy that there is a chance I can help you. You're too young a man to have to live with pain for the rest of your life."

My mum's face had a glow to it that I hadn't seen in quite some time. She was absolutely in awe as well and quickly handed over the forty pounds that Sandy charged for the session.

"Will I see you the same time next week then?"

"Absolutely Sandy, we'll see you then."

We made our way back up the garden path towards our car, and my walking was vastly improved; so much so that my mother was struggling to keep pace with *me*.

"Where's the fire?" she said with a rosy glow on her face as I looked back at her.

"Hey, give me a break, I haven't felt like this in a while. I still can't believe what just happened there. It's a little spooky, but whatever works I suppose."

"Son, if it works, we keep doing it. Don't worry about the money. The main thing is we do what we need to do to make you better."

She meant every word of it as well, and would've done anything in her power to help me.

The healing effects from the session with Sandy lasted for about two days. After that point I gradually regressed to where I had been before. I would give it a chance though. Like he said, it could take a few treatments to get the most out of it and I wasn't about to give up on it now.

I continued paying Sandy a visit every week for the next month, but each time I was only getting a few days of relief before reverting back to my days of pain. I pursued it for a few more weeks, but at this time, the period of reprieve was getting shorter and shorter, and eventually I gave up on it. I had no doubt that he had a true gift, and it had been like nothing else I'd ever experienced, but part of me wondered how much it was mental relief on my side. At first I was in so much jubilation that there may be something out there that was going to actually help me, and perhaps the thought was so stimulating by itself, that the positive frame of mind it gave me could've been a contributing factor. As time passed by I could see that it wasn't the phantom cure I'd first hoped, as the duration of relief diminished considerably. It had been worth a shot, but it was back to the drawing board again as far as exploring further options to make me better.

Live or Die

Things were becoming worse, particularly the mornings—more so than ever before. When I awoke it felt like I'd been set in a plaster cast overnight, unable to flex any of my joints. I was fighting it, but I was losing the battle. I wanted to be dead. It was the one sure way of ending the pain and the life long struggle seemed more of a certainty than a possibility. I could hardly get out of bed though, never mind find the strength to do myself in.

This morning in particular was the worst I'd ever encountered. I literally was unable to get out of bed.

"STEVIE, STEVIE," I hollered at the top of my lungs. I needed some assistance. It must've been bad to take those measures as I was a proud guy who was determined to do at least the basics on my own. More to the point I was sleeping naked, and the prospect of another guy—friend or otherwise—helping me naked out of my own bed was a horrifying prospect. More to the point, the size of Stevie's manhood was no secret—it was about the size of a policeman's baton and about as thick as a can of Red Bull. He was well renowned for showing it off during house parties, particularly while he was wasted. I would've done the same if I'd had a trophy penis. In this case I didn't need the embarrassment of him viewing my inadequacies relative to his stature—but under the current circumstances I had no choice.

There was no reply. He had been out with his new chick Becky the previous evening and had likely spent the night in throws of passion around at her place. For once in his usual bachelor type lifestyle he seemed content with this girl and good luck to him.

I lay back and pondered—there weren't any other options. I thought of my imaginary teenage leukemia stricken friend.

Hang in there Brandon; it's going to be OK. Stay with me for now. I might not have much longer myself and I need a friend to talk to.

He was right. I had to stop being such a pussy and fight; treat this like a hangover when I was younger and fitter. Back then the affects of alcohol had prevented me from wanting to get out of bed some mornings.

I again thought about Stevie and how happy he'd become with Becky. I could sense this was more than a fling for him as his whole demeanor had changed. He was still the same old Stevie, and continued to act in his usual drunken and crazy ways, even in front of Becky, but there was a respect he showed her that I'd never seen before from him, and they often looked into one another's eyes in a way that spelled out LOVE. This was the real deal.

In a way I was jealous of him—and not just because of the size of his weapon, although that would've been a hardship I could've lived with! I wondered if I would ever get the opportunity to experience those feelings for a woman again. Who would want this though? Who the hell would want to wake up beside their guy and have to help him out of bed, put on his socks and tie his shoelaces for him? The latter being a current exercise I had to leave myself an extra fifteen minutes in the morning to take care of before heading wearily to the office.

Around three months before, I'd been seeing a lovely girl by the name of Liz. She was separated from her husband and had two lovely kids. Initially it was just a sex thing with her. I'd met her one evening at the local bar when the alcohol had taken effect on me and limbered up my joints not to mention a pain killing effect also.

My friends and work colleagues Robbie and Anthony had began talking to her while her date for the evening had slipped off for a quick piss. They were being overly direct with her as they were drunk, but from previous experiences, Anthony was just the same even when sober.

"So do you like this guy?" questioned Anthony to Liz, pointing towards the men's bathroom door.

"He's alright, but it's our first date," replied Liz, being a little coy, but from her suggestive body language I could tell she was a frisky one.

"What do you think of our friend?" asked Robbie signaling towards me, no messing around.

This was a risky topic to bring up, as the guy in the bathroom was surely washing his hands by now. They asked her as though I wasn't even there or at least out of ear shot, but I was right beside them and becoming more uneasy by the second.

"He's cute," she said, opening up a little as she eyed me up and down, but one eye was wary of her date arriving back.

"That's settled then, give him your number and you can have a first date with him tomorrow," piped in Anthony as the bathroom door opened and her date reappeared looking a little rattled at seeing three strange guys around his woman for the evening.

I was over the moon that she'd described me as cute and even more delighted when I surveyed her date for the evening in more detail. He was a frail-looking smallish guy, not unlike my current condition. Maybe I was someone's type after all. He was very timid as he sat down, and Anthony brazenly introduced himself. He returned the gesture stating his name was Mike.

"This is Robbie and Brandon," said Anthony.

"How you doing?" said Mike, rather tentatively and confused, probably wondering what the hell was going on.

"Liz and I used to work together," lied Anthony, which seemed to settle the little dork down a notch.

Anthony was a very intimidating person to the eye, but was a bit of a teddy bear when you got to know him. He was a giant—probably around six feet six in height, and as confident as a stand-up comedian in front of a boisterous audience. Mike was certainly intimidated, and there was no doubt in my mind he wouldn't openly question where they'd worked together, not until Liz and himself left the bar, but by that time she would likely have a story straight in her head.

Liz was enjoying this in a way, obviously finding us *way* more entertaining than Mike had been towards her, and was giving me a few sultry glances as Anthony locked Mike in conversation about what he did for a living.

By this point we had moved our chairs from the adjacent table and were now cozily located beside Liz and her little geek. The interior of the bar was a typically traditional looking English establishment. The ceiling was lined with wooden beams and there was wood burning in the fireplace in the corner, enabling folks a comfortable escape from the cold and wet weather outside. To me this was genius on behalf of the bar management. The fire gave it a homely feel, and who would want to quickly leave such an environment to venture outside on a dreary, chilly evening? So why not stay for another pint of bitter and perhaps a shot of whisky to warm the cockles.

Robbie and I were finding our form with Liz; our comments littered with suggestive double entendres that were in turn increasing the rate of seductive looks towards me.

Liz was a good looking woman, obviously no stranger to the local gym. Her arms were tight and although she was dressed in a pair of tight black pants, they hugged her curves enough to tell she was firm all around. Her hair was blonde, but obviously straight from a bottle, as her dark roots were beginning to peek through, and I couldn't help my mind from wondering whether the carpet matched the curtains! She was in my book about a seven out of ten. She'd never make the cover of Vogue magazine, but then again I would never be challenging for a spot in Beach Body Monthly, but her personality was an absolute treat. She almost came across as being "one of the boys" in the way she spoke about the local soccer club, as well as how she enjoyed a good drink, and had a mouth on her like a sailor—an attribute many men would have found a turn off, but I wasn't one of those men.

An hour or so passed and Anthony was buying drinks for all of us like prohibition was just around the corner. As he headed to drain off the six pints he'd consumed, I decided to follow, as I wanted to know what he was scheming—there was certainly something. Also, I didn't want to be left talking with just Liz and Mike, as I was sure if I hadn't pursued Anthony as quickly as I did, then Robbie would've been right on his tail. It would've looked extremely weird if the three of us had gone at the same time—two was socially acceptable, three was just plain creepy. That was an unwritten rule.

"She's a bit of alright." said Anthony towering above me only two urinals away.

"Yeah, she's cool as shit. What you up to?"

"*Me?*" he replied, with a smirk and a look of guilt that any lawyer couldn't have debated against.

"Yeah you. You know what I'm talking about."

"I'm trying to get you hooked up with this tasty bit of gear. She looks like she's mad for it. I just wish I was a single man again. I'd be in there like a ferret up a drain pipe."

Both Anthony and Robbie were married. They could tell I was struggling every day at work and no doubt aware I wasn't seeing much action in the loving department.

"So what's the big plan then?"

"I'm trying to fill everyone with beer. The little boyfriend fella's just been for a pee about an hour ago, but from the looks of him he's not the sort who can handle any serious quantity of alcohol, so hopefully he'll be back in here shortly. Robbie can join him for distraction purposes, just in case he tries to squeeze it out quickly and come back to the table without washing his hands. No doubt he'll be a bit wary of his chick getting a bunch of attention, so he'll try and get in and out in double quick time. While that's going on Liz can write down her digits for you and BOOM, you'll be nostril deep in inner thighs by this time tomorrow evening."

"You've got it all worked out don't you."

"I *am* the master."

"What if she doesn't have a pen or paper?"

"Way ahead of you chief," he said pulling a napkin and pen from his back pocket. "I swiped these from the bar while I was up getting the last round in."

I had to respect his attention to detail, but wasn't fully convinced it would go down quite as smoothly.

We arrived back at the table. Liz had a bored look on her face, but perked up with a saucy smile as we appeared from the bathroom. Mike had Robbie involved in some form of conversation, but my good buddy looked like he was losing the will to live. That was the precise reason I had to join Anthony in the bathroom. The beer was slightly warming Mike up and I didn't want to be the one landed talking to him, as there might be no escape, and I wanted all my time and attention focused on the lovely Liz.

"Another round then?" inquired Anthony, fully refreshed from his pee that any horse would've been proud of.

"Maybe we should get going," said Mike to Liz.

"We can stay for one more," she replied, which was music to my ears.

She was way out of his league and he knew it, so didn't provide much resistance to her wishes. He didn't want to blow it with her already, but in my mind he already had.

One drink turned into three and I could tell young Mike was ready for a bathroom break as I could feel the vibration of his dancing leg as it bounced against the table. He seemed reluctant to go, much like Anthony had suggested. It was just a matter of time though. Pissing himself would certainly be an end to the evening, so better to take the gamble on a visit to the restroom.

As he opened the bathroom door, Mike gave a final look back at our table, and he almost had an expression of surrender on his furrowed brow. No sooner had the door closed behind himself and Robbie; Anthony produced the pen and napkin.

"So you gonna give Brandon your number?" he said, sliding the pen and paper across the table to her.

"You guys are terrible," she replied, half heartedly as she scribbled her digits and passed me the napkin, which I quickly folded and slipped into my back pocket.

"I'll give you a call tomorrow," I said, looking deep into her eyes.

"I'd like that," she replied, enthusiastically returning the gaze.

Our timing had been impeccable, as Mike appeared only a few seconds after the exchange. I felt sorry for him for two reasons. Firstly, it was maybe a little out of order to go behind a guy's back and hit on his date, but she could've said no, so that neutralized the guilt from my end. Secondly, even with Robbie present, he'd obviously hurried his piss along at an alarming rate and neglected to give his penis the necessary number of shakes when he was done, as there was a small coin shaped wet patch clearly visible on the outside of his pants near the crotch. It wasn't even located much below the end of his zipper, indicating he wasn't particularly well endowed either!

"You ready to go?" asked Mike with a hint of desperation to his tone.

"Yeah," said Liz, quickly gulping down the remainder of her drink.

"Well it was nice to meet you both," I said.

"Yeah, take it easy," said Anthony, trying his best to hide the smirk on his face.

"See you later," said Robbie, also fighting a smile.

"Thanks for a good night guys," replied Liz enthusiastically, as they made their way out of the bar and back into the windy and cold elements.

The three of us laughed heartily.

"You gonna give her a call?" inquired Robbie.

"I'd be an idiot not to."

"Yeah you would. She was well tasty," said Anthony, grabbing his balls.

I was looking forward to the call with Liz tomorrow. A bit of female companionship was just what the doctor ordered (not literally of course). I was almost positive that tonight would be Mike's first and last date.

"Hello."

"Liz?"

"Yes."

"Hi Liz; it's Brandon from the bar last night."

"Hi Brandon; I was thinking about you this morning and hoped you would call."

That was music to my ears, and gave me a little confidence boost; something that I'd been lacking for a while.

"Yeah, I was thinking about you as well. What you up to?"

"Not much, just doing a bit of housework at the moment, the kitchen's a bit of a bomb site. What about you?"

"Nothing much, just having a bit of a lazy day so far. I'm meeting a buddy for a beer this afternoon and maybe a couple of games of pool, but other than that I don't have any plans."

"Would you like to come over tonight and I'll cook you some dinner?"

"That sounds great."

"Maybe around seven?"

"That works for me."

"You got a pen and paper so I can give you directions?"

"Yes I do; go ahead."

Fortunately I still had the same pen and napkin from the previous evening, and I eagerly scribbled down the details.

I pulled up at the address around ten after seven; I didn't want to be over punctual and appear a little too keen. Liz lived in a nice looking neighborhood; the streets quiet and populated with well kept semi-detached homes.

I was a little edgy inside as I made my way to her front door. The garden was neatly manicured; the tightly mown lawn enclosed by an array of beautifully trimmed flowering shrubs, so I was sure the interior of the house was equally as pristine—especially as she was expecting company.

I confidently knocked the stained glass door with three rhythmical beats. Through the door I could see a curvy silhouette rapidly approaching.

"Hi there, I'm so glad you could make it," said Liz, followed with a glowing smile that only further brightened my already cheerful mood.

"I wouldn't have missed it for the world," I replied, giving her a wink.

"Come on in."

"Thought you'd never ask," I said in a sarcastic tone.

"I can see you're going to be trouble," replied Liz with a chuckle.

We exchanged a kiss on the cheek and I followed her in the direction of the living room. She looked ravishing, and there was even more sexiness to her than the previous night. Her legs were on display as she was sporting a red cotton miniskirt. My attention was swiftly brought to her long sleeved black t-shirt style top. The front had a printed picture of two melons, and the word "JUICY" was written underneath. It was a little tacky, but a more than adequate description of her perky and tasty pair, and only added further fuel to the fire on my thoughts of her being a frisky one.

"Nice place you've got here."

"Thanks, but it doesn't always look this organized."

"I'm sure it does compared to my place."

"Probably, but all you guys are slobs."

"Well I'm not going to disagree with that."

"I hope you like Spaghetti Bolognese."

"Sounds wonderful."

"Good; either that or we'd have to order pizza or something."

"No, I love Bolognese."

"Cool; do you wanna eat now or just hangout for a bit first?"

"To be honest, I could eat right now, I'm starving. I've been saving myself all day for this."

"Glad to hear it. Grab a seat at the table and help yourself to some wine. I'll be through in a couple of minutes with the food."

"Perfect."

She made her way out of the room and I followed her every move. Her ass fitted the skirt like a tight glove and her calf muscles were perfectly toned.

I poured us both a couple of glasses of red wine. Liz had obviously gone to a lot of effort. The table was decoratively covered with a satin style table cloth, the best cutlery had been pulled out for the night, and two red candles stood tall in a Victorian style silver holder, perfectly dissecting the two place settings. I removed the cigarette lighter from my pocket, lit the candles, and adjusted the dimmer switch on the wall in a vain attempt at creating some romance. I really should've brought her flowers, but I was never really the type unless I'd been a "bad boy" and needed to enhance an apology for being an asshole.

There was a real cozy feel to her home. It was small, but quaint, and was fashionably furnished with a beige colored leather sofa, dark blue carpeting, and the central heating was cranked up in an effort to combat the cool outdoor temperature.

Back she came, balancing two heaped plates of Bolognese, being careful not to spill any. Her steps were slow and deliberate, and had the precision of a trained tightrope walker.

"Let me help you with those."

"It's OK, I'll just end up dropping them if I try and hand them to you."

"This looks great," I said, as she placed them on the table.

The smell of garlic was fantastic, and the fact we were both eating it didn't worry me should any kissing occur before the evening was over.

Our conversation flowed with ease and I was sensing a real connection. Three quarters of the wine was already gone and Liz's cheeks had developed a rose-colored glow to them. I could tell she had a little buzz going as she laughed more enthusiastically than ever at my general goofiness.

"We've put quite a dent in this bottle," I said, topping up our glasses, and the remainder of the wine was gone.

"Holy crap, I wasn't even paying attention. Time flies when you're having fun I guess," she said with the sweetest of smiles.

"I agree. Listen, thanks for inviting me over, I'm really having a nice time."

Our eyes locked together and we held a stare that created such a pause that it was verging on awkward.

"Anyway, let me get these empty plates cleared up. Make yourself comfortable in the living room and I'll grab us another bottle of wine."

"You trying to get me drunk or something?"

"Maybe I am," she replied seductively, and headed through to the kitchen.

I sank perfectly into the contours of the leather sofa and gazed around the room as a way of distracting myself from the obvious flirtation between us; the last thing I needed was to get over excited at the prospect of something physical occurring.

Keep it together Brandon, you'll do just fine; it's like riding a bike. You never forget once you learn.

My heart was racing though and I was becoming seriously turned on. The inner tingling was firmly brought to a halt as I thought about my illness. Should I tell her now? There wasn't any point in that. We weren't involved in a relationship yet, so best to wait and see if anything developed first. It wasn't like I had some sexually transmitted disease or anything that would put her in jeopardy should we end up having some one on one fun. She had already asked me if I'd hurt my leg. I was having a great day in terms of pain level, but my limp was still very apparent. I blew it off with the old knee injury excuse and that it had flared up. It wasn't so much of a bare faced lie, more a slight bend of the truth.

Liz returned to the living room with a new bottle of wine and sat down beside me on the sofa. I took the new bottle and again topped up our glasses.

"Would you like to watch a movie or something?"

I wanted to respond "or something," and give her a wink, but that seemed a little forward and even presumptuous.

"That sounds cool; what you got?"

"Maybe something on pay per view; all my videos are really old ones."

"Perfect. Hold that thought though; I need to use your bathroom."

We both stood up and she pointed to the stairs.

"Straight ahead when you get to the top."

"Great, see you in a minute."

Again our eyes met, but this time something came over me and I moved in for a kiss. It was like slow motion as my face got closer, and she remained firm in her stance. Our lips met and we shared a soft but passionate embrace before I pulled away.

"That was nice. I've wanted to do that all night," I said, almost whispering.

"You have?"

"Yeah."

On that note I made my way to the stairs.

I hated stairs. Going up wasn't *too* bad. It was still sore on the bones, but slowly I could handle them if there weren't too many. It was coming back down that scared the crap out of me. The pain was significantly magnified, and I always had the vision of tumbling my way to the emergency room. It was weird why I tried to be alone as I shuffled my way down, but an audience sent my self-con-sciousness off the charts. Why should I care? I knew there was something wrong with me, but I always tried to appear as normal as I possibly could.

The trek up the stairs was trickier than usual in light of my current excited state. The kiss had caused a serious stirring in my pants and only added to my delicate steps as I made my way up to the bathroom. There was no guarantee that sex was on the menu, but it was looking like a serious possibility. I was consider-ably out of practice and an early arrival at the finish line was a distinct chance I had to take.

I washed my hands and face with cold water and stared in the mirror.

OK tiger, play it cool. Just relax; you've done this many times before.

I hurried as quickly as possible back down the stairs—still slow by normal folk's standards. I must've only left the living room around 2-3 minutes, but it seemed longer, and I hoped Liz didn't think I'd taken a dump; just in case she'd previously been considering going down on me.

"Thought you'd fallen in or something," she laughed.

"Really? I was only taking a pee as well. The old knee injury was just giving me a few aches and pains on the way down," I replied, making sure she was aware of which number I'd went to the bathroom for.

"No, I'm just messing with you."

"And you say I'm gonna be trouble," I said, sitting down beside her again and began frantically tickling her side and stomach.

Her laughter was verging on uncontrollable as I continued on, sliding my face in next to the right side of her neck. I stopped with the tickling and delicately placed a soft kiss on her cheek. I pulled back and we gave each other a gaze, noses no more than three inches apart. There was a momentary pause before we pounced on each other, kissing in a frenzy and tearing our clothes off like it was a race.

About fifteen minutes had passed—at least ten more than I'd envisioned, and we lay back on the couch panting, covered in sweat, with huge smiles on our faces, and we shared another kiss, soft and tender this time after our animalistic session.

"How was it for you?" I asked, half joking, but inside I was genuinely looking for feedback.

"Why do guys always ask that? How do you think it was?"

"I don't know."

"I thought the level of moaning and groaning I was doing would've been more than a subtle hint."

"I know, but us guys always like to hear some positives."

"Shut up and kiss me you crazy boy."

That night with Liz was something special and would always be part of my good memories.

We began seeing each other a couple of times a week after that night, each time becoming more passionate and connected than the previous occasion. As our bond developed though, I felt myself wanting to push her further away, even though deep down inside this wasn't the case.

I was having a bad day. The inflammation was hacking away at my knee joints like a lumberjack on an oak tree.

You'll be fine Brandon, just take a nice warm bath and smoke some dope and you'll be as good as new for your date tonight.

Even as the words were going through my head, I didn't completely believe them. There was no way I could let Liz see me in this state. We'd only been seeing each other for just over three weeks, and thankfully for me, each encounter had occurred at times when I was well enough to cover my illness with the old knee injury explanation.

Today was not one of those days. The burning sensation in my knees was intense, causing them to swell up like a couple of balloons, and the inflammation was steadily working it's way through my entire system, resulting in a stiffness across my elbows, shoulders, and even my neck. It was as though I was living in a butcher's freezer, becoming stiffer and stiffer as the minutes passed by.

Perhaps tonight was the night to come clean and lay my cards on the table, in the hope I pulled a royal flush, but the prospect of a negative reaction and ultimate rejection swiftly eliminated that as an option. I would let her know soon, but I was having fun right now and looked forward to our time together. Maybe it was no accident that my arthritis had died down in intensity on our previous meetings; an upbeat demeanor certainly seemed to have a positive impact on my condition. The mind was definitely a powerful beast, so perhaps this would continue on and put the disease into remission for a while. It was worth the risk for now; no point in messing with a good thing. It was time for that hot bath and soothing smoke.

I lay in the tub; the warm water doing its best to ease my struggles, and I sucked eagerly on my roll-up, inhaling hard to gain maximum benefit. I hated the fact I was relying on an illegal drug to fight my cause. I wasn't usually one for breaking the law for recreational purposes. It angered me that the government hadn't stepped in to regulate this product for medicinal use, particularly when it worked as an effective pain reliever and there were millions of people around the globe suffering chronic pain on a daily basis.

My guilt quickly evaporated as I took a massive final hit of the cigarette and extinguished it under the cold tap. I sank my head back into the water, lying fully stretched, using my elbows to prop me up enough so that my nose just peeked above the surface.

I wish every moment could be as peaceful and relaxing as this.

My head was fuzzy and my entire body felt completely limp. The burning sensation in my joints was fading fast and I wished I could remain like this forever.

I could afford no such luxury though, as I stared at my watch through my tainted vision. It was just after six o'clock and Liz was picking me up around seven. We were heading into town for some Indian cuisine, and part of me wished I'd passed on the cannabis, as I now had the munchies—big time!

I slowly and surely pulled myself up onto the edge of the tub, and delicately dragged my legs over the side and onto the soft towel I'd laid on the floor. I was feeling a little better, but the prospect of Liz seeing me struggling was really bothering me.

She really was a sweetheart, but I couldn't stop myself from feeling she deserved better. These thoughts may have been dumb on my part as I knew I was a good guy and would treat her well, but I was always going to have the mentality that I was holding her back. I hadn't even told her of my condition, and the prospect of *perhaps* doing it this evening was scaring the crap out of me, as I knew deep in my heart that I wasn't prepared for the possibility of rejection. In my mind it was better for me to end things sooner than later, before I became too emotionally attached.

She was an extremely active person; a regular at the gym, rode her bike for miles at the weekend, and generally enjoyed any high intensity exercise. Sure, we'd probably get on well for a while, but my idea of a long lasting successful relationship was one where you could share similar interests and enjoy time together. The future on that front did not look bright. I'd end up being the proverbial ball and chain around the ankle, dragging her down and eroding away her zest for life. It had to end; there was no other way.

The doorbell rang right on schedule and I opened the door to the familiar glowing smile that I'd become extremely fond of.

"Hey sweetheart, how you doing?"

"Better for seeing you," she replied, planting a moist kiss directly on my awaiting lips.

"Thanks for the compliment; great to see you as well. I'm ready to go if you wanna get going?"

"We *could* go now, or I could come in for a little bit if you know what I mean."

"That sounds great, but I've a feeling the restaurant might be a little busy if we don't make a move right now."

"Well OK, but I'm gonna get you later," she said, giving me a sexy wink.

I wasn't one for turning down sex very often, but I was still in a little bit of pain and the prospect of rolling around frantically wasn't appealing at all, so I decided to lie as far as the restaurant being busy. It may have been, but I wasn't basing my statement on any known facts. I was also feeling rather guilty. I'd decided this relationship was likely going to end which ached me inside, as she really was a little gem, but I couldn't work myself past the inevitable frustration I would cause her further down the line.

We arrived at the restaurant and made our way inside. The décor was traditionally Indian with its colorful fabrics and wallpaper illustrating a huge map of India together with the key cities and landmarks elegantly highlighted. The level of detail shown for the Taj Mahal was particularly impressive. Even the female wait staff was clad in their long silk Sari outfits which were a special touch.

"So much for it being busy."

"I really thought it would be," I said almost embarrassed, trying to fight the possibility of blushing.

There were more vacant tables than not, and the hostess with the traditional Bindi on her forehead looked genuinely pleased she had a couple of extra folks to add to the current ambience.

"Your knee seems to be bothering you more than usual," said Liz with a concerned look.

"Yeah it is. Hopefully a few Kingfisher beers will help numb the pain," I replied with a chuckle.

Again with deflecting the subject. Come on Brandon, just tell her the truth.

We got comfortably situated in a cozy booth in the corner by the front window, looking out over the busy main street of the town. Several couples passed by hand in hand or with arms around one another. They all looked so happy and content together. I longed for a similar rapport, but I knew that was an unlikely future event. Perhaps I was destined for a life on my own. Maybe it was just the way it was meant to be. I did have to focus on myself, find a way to get better. Was I being selfish? There was a chance that I was, but I couldn't see any other plan of attack.

"Liz, I need to tell you something."

She had an almost alarmed look on her face as the words came out of my mouth. The tone used was obviously an easy indicator that I wasn't about to dish out some wonderful news.

"This sounds serious."

"It is. Look, I haven't been completely honest with you up until now."

The look on her face intensified.

"My story about the knee injury wasn't exactly true. I've had my share of knee knocks over the years, but it's a lot more serious than that. I was diagnosed with arthritis a while back and the knee trouble is a result of that. The condition affects most of my large joints like my knees, hips, elbows and shoulders. They get stiff and painful quite a lot at times. I have my good days and bad, but it's not something that's going to go away. If anything, there is a good chance I'm gradually going to deteriorate."

I knew it wasn't the case, but I almost felt like the noise level in the room had dropped a few decibels as a result of the confession. The initial look of shock on Liz's face had now been replaced by one of sympathy.

"Oh my God, you poor thing," was the only reply she could give.

She genuinely felt sorry for me as her eyes became very glassy in appearance.

"I suppose, but it is what it is. So if it bothers you, now is as good a time as any to jump ship. I'll fully understand and would never hold it against you."

"Don't be ridiculous, it's no big deal to me," she replied, trying to maintain as positive a tone as possible, but I could tell she now had a million and one scenarios running through her mind.

We ordered food, which was a nice interruption to the current situation, then we continued on as though nothing had ever been said, but the conversation was flowing as well as a river halted in its progress by a group of beavers.

I hated the fact she was feeling bad for me. I *didn't* want any pity, but as much as she was trying to conceal the fact, it was very evident she was doing a bad job of it. What was she really thinking? Was she picturing a scenario of having to cater for my every need further down the line? Maybe she was figuring out a nice and tactful way to break things off, without coming across as a complete bitch. I knew I was being over analytical and that my paranoia had kicked into overdrive, but I *was* feeling extremely uncomfortable with the present moment in time.

End it now. Beat her to the finish line.

My mind was working overtime as I lay back in bed staring at the heavens. Having trouble sleeping wasn't a surprise, but with all the turmoil spinning in my messed up head, I was as alert as alert could be. As much as I tried, I couldn't work my way through the awkwardness that had developed with Liz since my big announcement. I couldn't ask her the questions I wanted to as there was little chance she would've given me honest answers. Even if I did pose these questions, it would be exposing my weakness and vulnerability, which in my mind were never attractive qualities. Tomorrow was going to be tough, but it was the day to bring this torture to an end.

"Hi, can I speak to Liz please?"

"Yes, who's calling?" said the perky sounding office secretary.

"It's Brandon."

"One moment please."

I hated doing this over the telephone. Maybe it was the cowardly option, but my work day had been as productive as a dope head on a Sunday morning. I just couldn't focus on anything. I'd even tried taking extra break time in the smoking room and conversing with folks I barely knew, but I was like a deaf person unable to lip read. Their mouths were moving but nothing was registering; now had to be the time.

"Hi there," said Liz in a tone not filled with the usual cheerfulness that generally accompanied her greetings.

It could've been that she was having a rough day at the office, but my messed up mind interpreted it as a sign she was sharing the awkwardness.

"Hey, sorry to bother you at work, but I really needed to talk to you. I've been thinking a lot about dinner last night and my whole medical situation, and I don't think I'm ready for a relationship right now. I think you're a lovely girl and all, but I have *way* too many issues going on right now, and I think it would be better if we were just friends."

I was literally shaking, and it had an impact on some of my words which were delivered with an element of a stutter. There was an eerie pause before she finally responded.

"Well Brandon, I'd be lying if I said I wasn't disappointed, but if you feel that is what you need to do there's not much I can add to it."

"Unfortunately it is. I'd still like to stay in touch with you though and maybe hangout from time to time. Grab a drink or something."

"That would be nice."

"Well, take care of yourself and I'll be in touch."

"You as well Brandon."

I couldn't help but feel sad as I hung up the phone, yet relieved at the same time. Be friends, stay in touch, hangout, have a drink sometime. What a bunch of crap. Who was I kidding?

Talk to Me

What the hell are you doing? She was a fantastic girl. Maybe she didn't give a crap about your stupid condition. Maybe you just gave up on the one girl on this screwed up planet who was ready to accept you for who you are. OK, you're no beach babe muscle bound Adonis, and never will be, but those freaks are not everyone's cup of tea. Perhaps she saw someone in you who could stimulate her not only in the physical sense but mentally as well. Perhaps she was happy she could give up the gym membership and the boring ass bike rides that she struggled to endure. Maybe she thought her sleek tight body and defined calves and thighs were the expectation from us male scumbags and the only way of catching that prize winning salmon from the piranha filled lake; a sacrifice she was never delighted about having to pursue. Maybe she was finally happy she could throw away those so called vices that had been mentally dragging her down for a long time. Maybe you're not the only one who's been putting a brave face on things, living a life you didn't want to lead.

You could be right though in all that you are thinking. Maybe she was in a panic with the situation. Maybe she had all these future activities planned; skiing, rock climbing, mountain biking over tough terrain and endless Kama Sutra positions that only a medalist in the Olympic gymnast division was capable of achieving. What if she had high hopes of the soccer or martial arts background you'd talked about being put into training of future kids into MLS stars or UFC contenders? Yeah, you'd be a great help with that crippled boy! What if she'd actually wanted you to sign up for the joint membership at the gym and take advantage of the family price reduction? Oh yeah, that would've been wonderful. Watching you in eager anticipation out of the corner of her eye as she peddled at a ferocious pace on the exercise bike, disappointed that you were squatting about as much weight as the fat kid in class taking a dump; the one who was too scared to touch the toilet seat with his pimply ass because his sadistic older sister had told him he could potentially contract a dose of crabs.

The answers to these thoughts would never be discovered. Pride and principal of the actions already taken—rightly or wrongly—would prevent any further contact with Liz.

Visit Back Home

It was a cold winter weekend back in Scotland. I could certainly pick the weather for a visit back home. The wind howled like a distressed wolf, and the snow appeared to be falling horizontally. The trees were as bare as a baby's ass and offered no resistance or shelter from the blizzard-like conditions.

I slowly pulled into the hospital parking lot, being extra careful to trace the parallel tracks the vehicles before me had cut out in the ever increasing levels of snow. I was in enough pain and panic today, and the last occurrence I needed was straying from these indentations and potentially losing control and possibly causing further injury. Who knew if there was slippery ice under the powdered layer.

This was an emergency situation. The previous night my left knee had ballooned to the size of a steroid ridden grapefruit. This morning it resembled a normal shaped knee, but my left calf would've been at home on a champion weightlifter. Don't get me wrong, it was an attractive looking calf, but perched next to my little right chicken leg didn't take Dr. Gregory House to identify there was a problem. It was throbbing, almost visibly so with a heartbeat of its own. I may not have had House's number, but Dr. Marshall was already on speed dial.

I described my symptoms and he suggested I take myself to the Emergency Room ASAP. He said it may not be anything to worry about, but it was a *potential* indicator of a blood clot, and if so, and not attended to, there was every chance of losing the lower half of my leg. He may have been dramatizing a little to make sure he was covered, but the sheer mention of amputation had me scrambling for my car keys.

I called my mum on my cell phone as I broke the speed limit as much as the weather conditions allowed, and she was going to meet me at the hospital. Her office was close by, so I knew she'd be first to arrive. I deliberately didn't regurgitate the words from Dr. Marshall. One of us in a complete panic was more than enough.

The main roads were fine as the gritting trucks must've been out early in the morning, and I belted along, weaving in and out of traffic, horns sounding as I passed. Other motorists probably thought I was some reckless imbecile with no regard for road safety and weather conditions. If only they knew.

I was going to be able to get out of the car *fairly* close to the E.R entrance. For once luck was on my side as an elderly lady was pulling out of a spot next to the disabled spaces.

Come on, lady, I know these are difficult conditions, but get a move on.

She was as deliberate as a learner driver, being careful not to bump the car next to her, which was completely redundant as you could've hand brake turned a school bus into the space.

Eventually Granny Blue Rinse pottered her way towards the exit, consistently deviating from the furrowed tracks, which wasn't completely surprising as her seat was so far forward I was amazed she could even squeeze her frail frame into the car, never mind have room to enable unobstructed maneuvering. I could barely see her graying eyebrows peering over the steering wheel. If it wasn't for the puffy permed dyed hair job, you'd almost have thought the car was driving by itself.

I timidly made my way towards the E.R entrance. The ground below me was like a skating rink, and I was convinced a seasoned ice hockey player would've struggled with navigation, never mind a skinny arthritis riddled young man.

The snow flakes were flying towards me like a series of miniature ice bullets. It was just typical that I had to be walking against the wind and not with it; like I wasn't struggling enough. I could see the faint outline of my mother outside under the covered entrance way. I could make out a worried look on her face, in between being partially blinded by the incoming projectiles. I knew she wanted to come to me to aide my struggles, but she refrained, knowing I'd likely give a frustrated objection, citing "I'm fine, I can do it myself."

I always resisted assistance, which was essentially retarded. I *wanted* to believe I was normal and could climb K2 if I'd chosen to, but I was only kidding myself. I *was* a stubborn pig, something I needed to get over.

On this occasion a helping hand would've been a welcome one, but like any other time this realization registered in my thick skull, I'd still never ask or admit to it for that matter.

Finally the Arctic expedition was over, my face scattered with many circular red blotches. It was probably the first time in my life I'd wished my eyesight was as functional as my major joints. A pair of glasses would've certainly helped in deflecting some of the stinging pain.

"What's wrong, why do you need to be here? Is it serious?" said my mum, spitting out the panicked words at one hundred miles an hour.

"Can we go inside?"

"Sorry son, but I'm just worried about you. You were just so vague on the phone."

We made our way into the bland, washed-out looking lobby. I suppose the pale appearance of the room matched the overall mood, but surely part of the hospital budget could've been pushed towards a fresh lick of paint; swap out the over washed underpants blue with some summer yellow, orange, or red. Brighten up the place and maybe the mood would follow. Throw up a few decorations or scenic photographs. Give the ill or wounded something to look at while they waited in the line resembling that of the theme park rollercoaster ride on a holiday weekend. The status quo only added to the depression, and the waiting room had the get up and go atmosphere of the local morgue.

The Emergency Room was aesthetically sad, but also the characters filling the place were as equally full of life! Not that they should've been ecstatic, but you would've thought they were all dying. If their ailments had been immediately life threatening they would've been waived the additional pain of having to wait around in this lifeless environment.

A chubby woman with greasy black hair across from us wearing a leg brace was rocking back and forth in her chair, making a continuous low toned droning noise. I never doubted she was in pain, but was convinced that everything upstairs wasn't in full working order either. She definitely didn't carry the sharpest spear in the tribe that was for sure.

There were another two gentlemen in the corner that I singled out. Both were obviously intoxicated; their speech being loud and slurred. The Scottish accent can be a tough one for foreigners to comprehend, but even *I* was having difficulty deciphering every word on this occasion. Only the curse words were as plain as day. It wasn't hard to tell which of the two was here for medical attention; although they could've both legitimately put forward a case. The guy on the right was being held in an upright position by the back of his seat and the adjacent wall. He had a thick, blood soaked bandage wrapped ruggedly around his forehead area; no doubt positioned by his dirty drunken friend in the torn jeans and stained overcoat, such was the neatness of the application!

Twenty, thirty, forty minutes passed, and my agitation was spiraling out of control.

"Relax, they'll get to you soon," said my mother, obviously sensing my frustration.

"They should at least change the name of this place to the 'We'll get to you eventually' room. Emergency my ass; I've got a calf that Arnold Schwarzenegger would be proud of and I'm expected to be as calm and peaceful as a Buddhist monk!"

Finally after ninety agonizing minutes I was called, and fortunately my blood clot fears were quashed.

A serious of tests showed that a pocket of fluid in my knee had burst and drained down in to my calf area causing the extreme swelling. Deep down I was relieved, but it was one issue after another with my health and it depressed me. I was fed-up with the time I had to spend in doctor's offices, hospitals, and laboratories for blood work. If I was to extrapolate out for the rest of my life at this rate it would likely equate to a total of two years lost time sitting in these places. It made me sick to my stomach.

The Upward Spiral Revival

The Land of Opportunity

Life in England was good in relative terms. It wasn't too much different from Scotland in many ways. The typical day consisted of waking up around seven thirty, fighting the urge to keep my crippled ass parked in bed until the afternoon, and then try and loosen up for twenty minutes before finally dragging myself wearily to my feet. Then it was the struggle of showering and climbing into whatever clean clothes remained, then enduring a long day at the office, attempting to maintain a fine balance of:

a. Keeping my mind on the job at hand, and

b. Fighting my paranoia and feeling sorry for myself.

The two feelings were like a see-saw battle most of the time. I had to keep pushing myself mentally to keep option b) as far in the air as possible.

After work was essentially the same script in both countries; either a lazy night watching crappy TV to distract me from the pain, or a jaunt to the local bar to fill myself with Guinness to dampen the aches. Either way it was the same shit in a different place.

"I'd like you to attend a conference in Fort Lauderdale next week. It is for continuous improvement in the manufacturing industry and I want you to go and bring back some best practices for implementation," came the Birmingham drone from my department boss Shane.

He was an extremely nice guy, but his voice always sounded as though he was in a depression, even when he was telling a joke at a work night out.

The words, although unexpected, were like music to my ears. The idea of the dull and damp current surroundings being replaced by high humidity and glorious sunshine, palm trees, and fake perky breasts was a breath of fresh air that was working wonders on improving my fading spirits.

I exited the terminal building at Fort Lauderdale airport. The warm air hit me like a blow torch and I instantaneously broke into a sweat. I hailed a yellow taxi cab which halted abruptly beside my awaiting bags. An over enthusiastic Jamaican looking Rastafarian guy greeted me with a beaming white smile. How he could function in this heat with the woolen multi-color Bob Marley type hat covering his bulging dreadlocks was beyond me, but I figured growing up in hot conditions got you acclimatized.

"How ya doin' mon?"

"Pretty good chief."

"Is that an Eengleesh accent I detect mon?"

"Nah, Scotland," I replied as he loaded my case in the trunk and we headed on our way.

I gave him the details of my hotel and hoped he wouldn't stiff me with the cost of taking a longer than appropriate route.

"First time in Fort Lauderdale mon?"

"Yes," I said, immediately wishing I'd said no.

Perhaps that was his way of finding out if I knew my way around or not. By responding "yes" I'd basically given him license to take the scenic route and in turn many more unquestioned dollars in his pocket. The fact I was putting the fare on company expenses though didn't cause me much concern either way.

"Do you smoke mon?"

"Yes, unfortunately I do. Hoping to quit soon though."

"Well you can go ahead and light one up if ya'd like. Us Jamaicans like a good smoke as well if ya know what I mean mon," he said with a laugh resembling a pig, as a result of the snorting noise that was tagged on at the end.

It was common knowledge that many Jamaicans liked to smoke, and usually something considerably more potent than a Marlboro Light.

Unfazed by the "No Smoking" sign stuck to the back of the car seat, I sparked one up and inhaled deeply. It felt good, as it had been around twelve hours since my last one.

In stereotypical cab driver fashion he bombed out of the airport at break neck speed with little regard to other road users. I wondered if he even knew he had a signal light to indicate his next maneuver; instead deciding to go for the more bullying approach of moving into different lanes whether other drivers liked it or not. The only good thing was that this type of driving was a good indicator to me that he wasn't trying to stiff me for money. Seemed like he was trying to get the ride over with ASAP, and probably get back to the airport again for another juicy cab fare.

I gazed out of the open backseat window at the passing scenery. It was certainly different from what I was used to seeing, as I blew my smoke out into the humid air. The place was like a billiard table, flat as a pancake with almost no inclines to speak of. It was certainly exotic looking, and the palm trees were evident in their hundreds.

I'd been to Florida before, but never the south. The previous visits were to Orlando with my folks many years back, taking ourselves to the Disney theme parks and water rides. We'd taken several cab rides back then, and the one thing that amused me was that every single taxi, even the one today, had their orange "Engine Warning Light" glowing on the dashboard. To me this was a signal that something was wrong, but each and every driver just continued on their merry way as though it was no big deal. It wasn't a big deal to me either as long as I arrived safely at my destination. I didn't fancy having us breakdown in this heat, as I was already sweating like a Greek marathon runner.

We exited the highway and made our way in the direction of the beach. Wow, there was some serious money in this area. What did some of these people do for a living? It seemed that every multi-million dollar house backed onto a canal, and I figured that maybe it was mandatory to have a twenty foot plus boat parked outside. Holy crap, I couldn't afford the fuel for one of those things never mind the boat itself and the mansion style house; and I was on what I thought was a substantial annual salary!

I found it remarkable how hot it was. The sun was beginning to go down, but it still felt like it was in the 80's. I might have been in Florida before, but I never remembered it being like this.

We finally pulled up to the Marriott beach hotel. It was an impressive looking set-up; sandy beige colored building and looked as though there were at least fifteen floors. The drive up to the foyer was exquisite. It was a twisting and turning narrow driveway, palm trees lined tightly on either side like a regiment of trained marines.

It was certainly an expensive joint, and I was glad my company was picking up the tab.

There was a doorman clad in a pristine white outfit consisting of pressed trousers and a short-sleeved white dressed shirt with the Marriott logo stitched in red thread on the left chest area, and his name and photo ID badge on the right hand side. Bob Marley popped the trunk, and Jose the bellboy kindly opened my door before retrieving my luggage. He was a jovial looking Latin guy, extremely polite and good natured. It was either his usual demeanor or the fact he'd be receiving a few dollars tip for carrying my stuff a mere twenty feet from the cab to the hotel lobby.

The interior was not surprisingly plush, decked out with marble floors and gold colored hand rails leading up to the restaurant.

I quickly checked in, sneaking my way to the desk in front of a group of about a dozen Japanese tourists. If I'd been stuck behind those guys it may have taken an eternity to get my room key, as a result of the quantity of them, not to mention the potential language barrier they posed. Fortunately for me they had been distracted by the fabulous décor, and were busy snapping photographs with their fancy cameras, zoom lenses resembling more of a rocket launcher than a piece of photography equipment.

Even the elevator was extravagant. The marble floor theme extended even to there, with the mirrored ceiling and walls being a nice additional touch. This was probably not appreciated as much by any of the resident honeymoon couples, looking to grab a discreet unnoticed feel of each other in their eagerness to return to their room and begin the frenzy of animal passion. They'd be exposed in a busy elevator for all to potentially see; although for some, the risk of being caught was likely an additional turn-on.

My room was huge, consisting of two queen sized beds with floral patterned quilts; carpet so thick and soft it felt like you lost an inch in height as you walked across it. There was a little corner office set-up, complete with a carved mahogany desk, matching swivel chair, night lamp and complimentary stationary kit.

I randomly ditched my bags on the floor and escaped from the comfort of the air conditioning, sliding open the glass balcony door, again the warm air hitting me smack in the chops. It amused me how opposite this place was compared to what I was used to. Back home we had to go indoors to warm up!

The view was awesome. I was on the 14th floor, and it felt like it offered me a visual range *beyond* the horizon. Day was slowly turning to night, sounds of squeaking bugs becoming more evident as God's dimmer switch leisurely ramped down. Couples still paraded half naked on the smooth sand of Fort Lauderdale beach, paddling ankle deep in the warm ocean as they merrily skipped along hand in hand on their romantic journey.

Hunger rumbled in my stomach like the tell tale sign of an earthquake beginning, but I resisted all temptation to opt for the lazy room service option, instead deciding to go with the outdoor cabana bar I could see next to the pool from my crows nest vantage point. My aching body could've done with a rest, but I was in the mood for a few beers as well as the food. It would take my mind off my usual train of thought when I was all alone with nothing to do, and I didn't relish feeling sorry for myself.

The Haitian bartender was involved in what looked like a heated debate as I perched myself in the bamboo style chair beside the beer pumps. His adversary in this case was a chunky looking blonde girl at the very end seat. Her chest seemed almost like it was inflated, and it was occupying her shoulder-less mint green tank top more than adequately.

The seats surrounding the L-shaped bar were moderately occupied. Every second seat seemed to be taken. The reason for this empty, taken, empty, taken situation was the fact the place was filled with individual businessmen. Guys treated seating arrangements—particularly in a sausage festival situation—just as they did when taking a leak in a public restroom. Rule 1: never pee in the urinal immediately next to one in the process of being sprayed if there is another one vacant further away. Bar seating etiquette was no different.

Jean the bartender finally introduced himself and poured me a pint of black velvet Guinness. I was amazed that an Irish beer had traveled this far, but as I shortly discovered, the taste didn't travel quite so well.

Jean was not to be trusted. They say first impressions last, and his Jekyll and Hyde persona had me wary from the very beginning. His almost aggressive antics when talking with Miss Chunky were immediately replaced with the politeness of an aristocrat as he turned to serve me.

The pool side tiki bar was quaint and peaceful. Each of the surrounding palm trees were circled at their base by small blue tainted lights that pointed skyward, only emphasizing their magnificence in the surrounding darkness. The bugs continued to chirp like birds, slightly louder than the faint reggae music coming from the small radio behind the bar.

I sparked a cigarette and swigged on my cold bottle of Heineken—that had quickly replaced the overly sour Guinness—and stared blankly at the small TV screen perched high in the corner. It was showing American football; a game I was completely unfamiliar with and even more baffled by the use of the word "foot" in its title.

"Excuse me," came the gentle words from the right of me.

I turned my head anyway, but hadn't expected them to be directed at me.

"Hi, what can I do for you?" I replied.

The softly spoken words had come from the chunky girl at the end of the bar.

"I'm sorry to bother you, but is there any chance you have an extra cigarette? I don't smoke very often, but I like to have one now and again when I'm drinking."

"Certainly," I said as I walked the ten feet or so to where she was sat and lit it for her. She took a huge inhale.

"Thank you."

"Anytime," I said, and made my way back to my stool.

I loved the term "do you have an *extra* cigarette." I was generally a bit of a wise ass and had been tempted to tell her yes it was her lucky day, as I just happened to buy a pack of twenty one earlier in the evening, but I felt it would've been a little inappropriate, and in my experience Americans didn't always appreciate sarcasm.

"What's your name?" she asked, obviously as enamored with the football game as I was, and looking for some form of conversation to serve as entertainment.

"I'm Brandon."

"Nice to meet you Brandon, I'm Nikki. Thanks again for the smoke."

"You're welcome Nikki."

"You on vacation?"

"No I'm on business, attending a conference."

"That's nice. You from Ireland?"

"Scotland actually."

"Wow, I hear it's beautiful over there."

"It is, but it has its not so nice areas like everywhere else."

We continued the small talk for five minutes or so before I moved over to the seat beside her. She may have been a regular at the drive-thru window, but she had an extremely pretty face and a very sweet personality.

The beers continued to flow and our conversation turned more friends like than two strangers passing in the night. The subject approached the topic of boyfriends and girlfriends, and she seemed rather pleased with my status. It turned out she didn't have a steady boyfriend, but had been out on a couple of dates with Jean the bartender, which explained the dagger-like looks he was occasionally drawing me.

"Do you fancy going somewhere else for a couple of drinks? I've basically had enough of Jean. He's so possessive, even though we've only been out a couple of times. I really don't want to see him anymore."

"Sure, sounds good. I need to be up fairly early in the morning though, but you are more than welcome to come back to my room if you'd like and we can put a small dent in the mini-bar?"

It was maybe a little forward, but I didn't want to go out to a club or something and make a crazy night of it and feel like complete crap in the morning, although that was still a distinct possibility considering I'd neglected to order any dinner.

"That would be cool."

I actually just intended to have a couple of drinks with her, but should anything else develop I was completely fine with it, as her little chubby cheeks and warm personality had quickly grown on me.

I settled up the bill and we headed off to my room. Jean didn't say a word, but I could almost feel his laser-like stare tearing a hole in the back of my head as we made our way back to the main building. I didn't feel too bad, as he wasn't Nikki's boyfriend and she was done with him, but I left a healthy tip as a form of guilty compensation.

Our conversation dulled a little as we headed up in the mirrored elevator. I was thinking about what might occur when we got back to the room, and I had a funny suspicion she was on the same page, although she was starting to physically look drunk. She had a bit of a slow blink going, but the few words she uttered on the ride up were at least legible and not slurred.

I took three attempts to open the hotel door; nothing to do with the alcohol consumption. I could never figure out which way to insert the credit card key. There were only four possible combinations, but in my mind it was never clearly marked and it was usually pure luck if I got it right first time. Three attempts were almost inexcusable though, but I put it down to the distraction of perhaps "getting lucky."

Mini-bar prices were extortionate, but I was expensing the trip, so dwelled on it for less time than it took me to flip on the bedside lamp.

I pulled out a couple of Bud Lights; the selection not exactly to my delight.

"Make yourself at home!" I said in the most sarcastic of tones.

Nikki was already lying down on the bed, head propped up with a couple of the super thick pillows.

"I am," was her reply.

My earlier assumption about many Americans not getting the whole sarcasm thing was quickly justified.

I parked myself down beside her as we said the customary "cheers" and clinked bottles together. My dislike of light beer became quickly apparent. It's watery flavor did nothing for me, but Nikki quickly gulped half of it down like I'd handed her some liquid gold.

To my instant joy she finished off the Bud and snuggled in next to me, head buried deep into my right pectoral muscle; or what I had of a pectoral muscle. It was going well, until she started to snore! Nothing was going to happen tonight so I decided to follow suit and drifted off.

I awoke to an empty bed. She was gone. Not even as much as a goodbye or a note on the bedside table. My first notion was that maybe it had been a set-up and that I'd been robbed, but my laptop and wallet was still around and there wasn't anything worth stealing otherwise. Maybe she'd been drunker than I'd thought and woke up wondering what had happened or where the hell she was. Either way was fine, as I never saw or heard from her again.

The conference was as expected; generally dull with a few amusing highlights from a couple of seasoned guest speakers. Why they'd sent me here was completely baffling. There wasn't anything from the day that couldn't have been picked up via two hours internet research, but if they wanted to shell out three thousand to wine and dine me, then I was fine with it also.

We took an afternoon coffee break, or "networking session" as they so elegantly referred to it.

There *was* actually some networking going on. I met a group of folks from Illinois who invited me out to dinner and drinks, which beat hanging out alone, distributing "extra" cigarettes and beers, and waking up alone with the brief feeling of being robbed and violated!

A gentle breeze mingled through the diners of the outdoor beachfront restaurant as the mellow sound of Jimmy Buffett's Margaritaville in the background added a nice touch to the feeling of peace and tranquility. This was the life. Everyone in the group had a carefree look about them; a far cry from the stress and strain of daily corporate life.

The rhythmical sound of the waves crashing onto the shore reminded me of the background music that played during a recent massage. There was no doubt it had a relaxing quality; so much so I'd almost forgotten about my chronic illness. I was definitely beginning to believe that mood had a strong influence on pain levels. The less stressed, the more at peace, and the more jovial I was, definitely seemed to correlate with a decrease in pain. Right now I had no stress, was as much at peace with life as a devout meditation practitioner, and the feeling of joy was escalating as I sipped on my second Pina Colada—complete with miniature umbrella stick and cherry—and watched the full moon high above the white surf. I felt great, and my aches were nothing more than a minor irritation.

It turned out to be a fantastic evening and I was becoming ever fonder with such an exotic environment. It was certainly a major contrast to the dull, bleak and uneventful nights back in the UK.

The following day at the conference was even slower than the previous one, particularly the morning, but that was more a result of a throbbing head brought on by the overindulgence of cocktails at the beachfront bar.

Our first "networking" break was a welcome one, and felt long overdue. I darted straight for the large table set-up with drinks and snacks and wolfed down a bagel and cream cheese and wired into the hot pot of coffee in an attempt to curb the hangover.

"Hi Brandon, I'm Bob," said the tall, smart-looking man next to me at the table.

At first I wondered how he knew my name, but I quickly realized the name tags we'd been asked to wear were more than a give away! My headache *was* really causing me to be a little mentally slower than usual.

"Hi Bob; nice to meet you."

"You work in our UK office is that correct?"

"Yes I do, but I wish I was over here in the Fort Lauderdale branch. It's beautiful over here and the weather is an absolute dream."

"Well funnily enough, that's kind of what I wanted to talk to you about. I work at the Fort Lauderdale office and have an opening in my team for a continuous improvement manager. I've been hearing from a few people that that's your role over there and you've got a lot of experience in that area. Do you think that might be something you'd be interested in?"

I was more than surprised to say the least but was instantly intrigued.

"It's certainly something I'd consider."

"Well let's get together at the next break and we can have an informal interview to determine if you'd be a good match for what I have in mind. I'll meet you back here at the coffee, as no doubt we're going to need one to waken up after this next lecture," he said with a grin.

"Sounds good Bob; talk to you then."

What a turn up for the books. They do say that opportunity knocks when least expected and this was certainly a pleasant surprise.

The next speaker was discussing six sigma applications to reduce product development cycle time; a topic equivalent to popping a sedative just before bedtime.

I sat there in the audience as the pompous presenter waffled on about how awesome he was and how he'd solved *so many* problems using these techniques—blah, blah, blah. My mind was miles away though, purely focused on getting together some good job application examples of my own to provide Bob with, in order to fill him with confidence as to my suitability for the role he'd mentioned.

Prior to the beginning of the lecture I'd cornered one of the guys I knew from the Fort Lauderdale branch to see if I could get a little inside knowledge about Bob. The feedback was exceptional. He'd come across as a super nice guy and my confidence had been given a rather nice boost by the fact I had essentially been recommended to him. The word on the street was he was a great guy to work for and was thought of as one of the knowledge gurus of the organization. This component was particularly appealing as I liked to surround myself with people I could further learn from.

We met back at the coffee table as planned and I filled us each a cup; this time using the larger of the polystyrene options as Bob was looking particularly weary.

"That one was a real snooze fest," I said with a chuckle, handing him a hot cup.

"Tell me about it; might have been more entertaining watching paint dry!"

We convened in a small seating area in the corner that was labeled "Mobile Meeting Area." These business hotels always had some form of phase for what were essentially four chairs and a small table.

Bob ran me through the job description and asked a few technical questions, which I responded to in a way I thought was extremely effective, and his positive head nods were more than encouraging.

It lasted no more than fifteen minutes before we moved onto discussing life in Florida and his passion for taking out his boat for a trip down the intra-coastal waterway on weekends. It all sounded like a fabulous lifestyle.

"Well the job's yours if you're interested."

"Really?"

"Seriously. I've been looking for a suitable candidate for a while now and you're the first who's really been on the same page as me. I'm looking to fill the position ASAP. What do you think?"

"Well I'm a little in shock to be quite honest. I came over her to pick up a few ideas for possible implementation projects back in the UK. The last thing I was expecting was a job offer and the prospect of moving across the Atlantic."

"Well take your time. I want to fill the position quickly, but I can wait a few weeks before that happens. It's been a couple of months already so another few weeks isn't going to kill me. I'd rather wait for the right person than fill it quicker with the wrong person. Why don't you chew it over and give me a call from the UK next week and let me know your thoughts?"

"Thanks Bob that would be great. I think I need a couple of days anyway to digest the idea and what it's going to mean to me."

"Not a problem. Here take my card and I look forward to hearing from you."

And that was that. He went on his way and I was left standing open-mouthed almost in disbelief. I had a lot of thinking to do.

The remainder of the conference came and went in an almost accelerated pace as my mind raced considering all the options I had. Even the flight home had my brain on overdrive which was unusual on long flights. My usual M.O was to throw down a couple of beers and watch about half of the in flight movie before dozing off and waking up as we descended; my shirt collar covered in drool.

This was not the case on this occasion as my brain was working overtime. The prospect of moving to the United States was an exciting one. I'd heard so much over the years about it being the land of opportunity and that there were healthcare options not available back in the UK, which was a major attraction for someone with my condition. Now was certainly as good a time as any as I had no relationship ties holding me back. It would be a tough decision to make, but one I would have to make sooner than later.

Days passed and it was all I could think about. I weighed up the positives and negatives, but there were very few of the latter other than the separation from family and friends. They could always visit, and I was sure that would happen frequently as they could treat it as a pleasant vacation as well as spending some time with me. I could also visit home from time to time. It really wasn't too far removed from my current circumstances anyway. Driving home to Scotland from the south of England could often take over six hours. The flight from Fort Lauderdale to Glasgow was under eight hours. It might cost a few extra bucks, but essentially there wasn't too much of a difference as far as travel time. I had no doubt my family would be more invigorated about visiting me at a sunny, exotic, palm tree clad destination rather than bleak and dingy Swindon and my corresponding crap hole of a home.

Decision made; it really was a no brainer.

A New Beginning?

Would this turn out like everyone had hyped it up to be, or would it be another link in the chain, similar to my Scotland to England transition—same shit different place?

Stop being such a complaining and pessimistic little girl and just get on with things. Move on, it's done now. If it doesn't work out, just go back home, but quit with the juvenile amateur dramatics. The heat might genuinely help your scabby excuses for joints.

That's what everyone told me before I moved over.

"The heat will do your joints the power of good," they would all say.

I never challenged their statements, but whether they were basing this on scientific evidence or it was just the fact this was a location where thousands of arthritic old aged pensioners settled in escaped me. Nice to be lumped in with the oldies if that was the real foundation of their well wishes!

It's not just an old person's disease!

So far things were not bad. Nothing mind blowing, but unique in many ways. It certainly was a different place, but same shit it wasn't.

My company had me set-up in a pre-paid apartment for three months; enough time for me to find my feet and bearings.

The biggest initial negative was that I was essentially all alone, which was never a good situation for my spiraling out of control mind. Friends and family were a continent away, and even although I could call and chat, my worst periods of negativity occurred in the lonely evenings after the tiring working days were over. The time in the UK is five hours ahead of Florida, meaning evening calls from my end were not an option. It would've been extremely selfish on my part to wake my folks up at an ungodly hour, just so I could vent. It wasn't like it was an emergency situation, and although they would've been more than happy to talk during my times of strife, regardless of the hour, it would've only led to *additional* worry for them that was *already* off the charts. It was better to portray a positive façade during the times we did talk.

I became quite the skilled actor during our conversations, switching my down beat mood into a positive sounding tone as soon as I dialed their number.

"Things are going great."

They were OK, but great was a stretch to say the least.

"The knees are much better. The heat really seems to be helping them."

Utter crap. I'd found the temperature had limited positive impact.

"Yes, I'm getting out and about, and I've got a bunch of new friends already."

True if two counted as a bunch!

Regardless of the truth or lies, my folks seemed more content, and believed that the move had been for the best. They missed me and still worried like crazy, but they were coming to terms with the geographical change.

The lonely evenings were quiet and uneventful. The only form of conversation was times when I had to consult with my teenage leukemia stricken friend.

Keep hanging in there Brandon, you know you can. The fact you're calling for me tells me you want to beat this.

Our little imaginary pep talks usually resulted in tears streaming down my face. The guilt, the fact I *was* actually relatively lucky, and he was lying there, bald little head not through choice, brittle looking frame, and his life clock ticking closer and closer to the point of no return.

My two friends were Robbie and Declan. Robbie had arrived out in Florida about a year before me, and we'd get together on work breaks at times, often recollecting stories from back in the UK, the incident of meeting Liz being our clear favorite.

Declan—or Dec as he was known—was an Irish lad who'd been in the United States since around the same time as Robbie. We all worked for the same company, and all became fairly close right off the bat.

I would go out with the guys, once, sometimes twice per week. It was generally nothing flash, just a few beers at the local British owned watering hole not far from the office.

The King's Head pub was a quaint little setting. It only held about sixty people max, but its wooden carved bar, a couple of slot machines, and an array of beer pumps with British logos on them gave it the authenticity of any traditional bar back in northern England.

I often called it "little Britain" as the clientele were mostly ex-pat implants wanting to recapture some of the homeland spirit.

I was comfortable at that bar. It was the one public place I lost all feeling of self-consciousness. Robbie, Dec and myself used to find a corner table, and generally either the boys got the drinks in, or the regular barmaid, Stella, would provide us with top quality table service. Regardless, I didn't have to expose myself and limited physical capability too often. The comforting fact for me though was that even when I'd take the short trip to the bathroom or rare venture to the bar, most of the stereotypical UK patrons were generally too inebriated to even pick up on it. Even if I crossed paths with another customer on my way up the short corridor to the restroom and they noticed my slow progress and limp, they just gave me a little wink and a "how you doing," indicating to me that they assumed it was a result of being just as drunk as they were!

Being in my comfort zone was important to me. The King's Head enabled that in a social setting, and it was the one thing permitting the release of built up frustration from a life that otherwise felt like a form of house arrest.

Stella made the bar though, and the fact her name was the same as the popular Belgian beer was additionally amusing considering her profession of choice. It was like it was meant to be, and just like a Jim I knew who worked at a local fitness club.

Stella was a real trip; super cheerful and always had a new joke up her sleeve every time she brought a round of drinks to our table. They were generally really cheesy, but we always got a kick out of them anyway.

"English guy goes to the doctor, drops his trousers and says, doctor, I've got a lettuce leaf sticking out of my arse. Doctor says, you've got more problems than that, that's just the tip of the iceberg," was one of her favorites. What made it even funnier was how she would crack up at her own joke, especially as she had obviously told it twenty times to other customers earlier that day.

She was a real looker for a forty year old woman, and just like Jim, was no stranger to a workout. It was like she dressed for tips. The tight denim shorts and low cut t-shirt exposing her washboard abs, and flirtatious manner, no doubt had a few of the clientele running to the bathroom at times for more than a number one or two!

Her short bleached blonde hair was an acquired taste, but certainly cute. It wasn't a style though that many females could pull off. It was like Sinead O'Connor and her shaved head—she actually suited it, and many guys would have lustfully mauled her in a heartbeat, but as soon as Brittany Spears decided it was a great idea, many of us thought she now looked as enticing as Shrek wearing lipstick and a mini skirt.

Stella had the ears for it though; small dainty things resembling baby ears, rounded on top and delicious looking little lobes. So many women, perhaps a result of a midlife crisis or something, would have their long flowing locks sheared off like a summer time sheep, only to expose that they really belonged on the planet Vulcan!

Robbie was probably the most sensible of us three stooges—although he had his moments—and was generally the designated driver the majority of the time, opting for only two or three beers, compared to the eight or nine that was common practice for Dec and myself. After he'd drop me off in my drunken state, back at the darkness of my company owned apartment, my mind would go into a thought process of a completely different dimension.

What would the scene be like if a super powered microscopic camera was sent into my knee joints? Would you see little termite looking creatures? Were they happily munching on my already depleted cartilage? Maybe they were in their own little contented world, merrily yapping away between their three square meals a day. Did they know what damage they were doing? They probably did.

Die termites, die.

After sobering up I knew I was letting my mind become over creative, but something was causing the joint erosion. Regardless of what the real scenario looked like, hope could be on the horizon. I had my first appointment in two weeks with my new rheumatologist, so maybe she was going to suggest a course of action that would make my latest beginning a new one after all.

I Love Your Accent

Life in the USA was generally good. The warm temperatures of South Florida perhaps *were* having a strange soothing effect on my joints after all. Maybe I just hadn't given it a chance to kick in and acclimatize my mind and entire body. The number of severe pain flare-ups had certainly decreased in comparison to the frequency they appeared back in the howling wind and cold of the UK. At least I could now genuinely respond positively to my mum when she asked if the heat was helping, as opposed to my usual bare faced lies. Although this was a glimmer of a positive, I still felt empty inside.

There was nobody here for me. My family and friends were all back in Scotland and England, making for many lonely nights—nights generally spent reflecting on life and questioning my decision to move across the Atlantic Ocean.

Real friends were few and far between. There was Robbie, but he had his wife and four kids, so I couldn't expect him to always be there for me during my moments of strife. There was Declan, who was in a similar position to myself—single, and his family and friends were back in Ireland. I wasn't ready though for painting the town red three times a week, as was the life Dec was leading. I was *so* self-conscious about my appearance and my lack of ability to walk normally, limping around as though I had a shoe full of gravel, and I could sense the people over here staring at me as they did back home, wondering what was wrong. It may have been lonely avoiding social interaction as much as possible, but it was better than the mental anguish the peering eyes caused me. I didn't want to lay all my issues on Robbie and Dec either. They had their owns lives and their own problems just like everybody else.

My weight was down to 106 lbs. I *looked* sick, which was only reiterated every time I took a single step. My face was gaunt and my cheek bones protruded like a skeleton on display in a city museum, and my Adam's apple felt like it stuck out like an actual real sized apple.

To many I looked anorexic; I could feel it, even though they would never say so directly. I *wanted* to eat, but the pain had a weird neutralizing quality that removed the urge. Maybe folks wondered if I had AIDS. This was likely my paranoia kicking in yet again, but to contract that virus required sexual contact which wasn't exactly breaking down my door right now and demanding some action.

It was a Friday evening as I sat watching TV in my second floor apartment, which had become almost a daily ritual. My place was very spacious, with an outdoor balcony that looked out over the pond of the apartment complex. As roomy as it was, it was equally untidy, and a thin film of dust covered the TV, VCR and every lamp shade around the place. I struggled to dress myself most mornings, so general housework and cleaning weren't even on my agenda. I really needed to invest in a maid though—even if it was only once per week.

The balcony though was my escape route to the warmth of the outdoors while still managing to avoid human contact, which was always a bonus.

I sipped on a piping hot cup of coffee as I watched the Howard Stern show. One of the commercials during the break was for a local chat line number. "Call and connect with other local singles in your area" was their slogan, and "first time users can try for free." I always thought these methods of meeting people were a bit sad and dripping with desperation. Perhaps so, but my existence was already sad and verging on desperate.

I contemplated with myself for a while, picking up the dust covered cordless telephone receiver before putting it down again. This cycle of debate continued for around ten minutes. It was like the process of calling a woman for the first time if she'd given you her number in the bar the previous evening. I was timid and rehearsing what to say, as I didn't know what to expect and worried about possibly make a complete ass of myself.

Finally logic hurdled my doubts. This was actually a perfect option. I needed more human interaction; I couldn't go on the way I was. This alternative was ideal as any ladies would never have to see me in my current state!

The process turned out to be an easy one, as I received my hour of free time. I recorded my name—using the fake one of Gary—and was prompted to provide a description of myself and what I was looking for.

"I'm Gary, a twenty-seven year old professional white male standing six feet tall with short dark hair. I'm new to the area, have a variety of interests, and looking for fun, outgoing ladies who like to laugh and are looking to chat."

In a small way I felt a little bad for giving a deceptive physical description. Shit, I wouldn't be six feet tall wearing a pair of clear stripper heels. It was very likely though that most people were bending a few truths. That was one of the luxuries of an anonymous telephone line; you could essentially be who and what you wanted to be. They couldn't all be attractive; otherwise I would've doubted they needed the phone line. How was I supposed to introduce myself anyway?

"Hi, I'm Brandon, a sad, lonely, anorexic-looking short ass Scotsman with a lack of friends, verging on depression with a serious lack of self-confidence. I'm seeking hot, confident girls with a fetish for skinny, mentally challenged guys with a strange accent, and who enjoy engaging in fun chat and occasional romantic candlelit dinners, as long as you promise not to look at me."

Yeah right, that would go down like a lead balloon and have them running for the hills.

I entered the chat line and began listening to ads. Navigation was easy; press one to request a live connection, two to leave them a message, or three to skip to the next caller.

I skipped through for a while. There was a real mixed bag of folks. Many were looking for their soul mate, others just some chat like me, some were plain freaky wanting phone sex or verbally simulating they were already playing with themselves, and others seeking "generous" males looking to meet right there and then, obviously soliciting an actual sexual encounter. I suppose it was a safer option for hookers than hanging around street corners in some dodgy neighborhood.

My eyes were certainly opening, and being given an insight into people's worlds behind closed doors.

The idea of having phone sex with a complete stranger had never really crossed my mind before, although it certainly was now. I painfully hobbled over to my patio windows and drew the vertical blinds, coughing profusely in the process as a cloud of dust filled the air as they closed, and attacked the back of my throat. A good dusting was what my apartment needed. The blinds had to be drawn in case I decided to indulge in some erotic phone play, and didn't need to provide any of my neighbors from across the small pond with an evening of voyeurism, as I participated in some hot talk with my pants around my ankles.

That could wait though, as I needed to build up some confidence with regular conversation before taking it to another level.

"Hi Pauline, I'm Gary; twenty-seven, six feet tall and new to the U.S. all the way from Scotland. You have a very cute sounding voice and I liked your description. Get back to me if you'd like to chat."

I hit the number four button to send the message and continued to scan through the other callers, hoping Pauline would get back to me.

Pauline, or whatever her real name was, described herself as having blonde hair and blue eyes with an athletic figure; five feet six in height and weighing about 115 lbs. She said she enjoyed the outdoors and long walks on the beach, and was seeking an active, fun, professional male looking for some intellectual conversation.

Perhaps she did have blonde hair and blue eyes, but when women felt the need to mention their weight I was always a little skeptical, particularly over the phone in this case. The likelihood was I could add at least ten pounds in order to arrive at the true number.

Many of the female ads stated they enjoyed the outdoors and long daytime walks on the beach, which puzzled me. I'd been to the beach on several occasions, and the folks there just lay around like they were dead, soaking up the golden rays from the Florida sun, not hiking along miles of beachfront in temperatures hitting the 90's. Maybe she meant at night or something, but I figured it was just a big bag of bullshit to appear hip.

The next few descriptions were rather disturbing. One was looking for an "open minded" male to go over for a "night of fun" with her and her husband—I quickly pressed the number three button.

The following "female" sounded anything but; voice as deep as Barry White and I had no doubt had an Adam's apple the size of a grapefruit (maybe the only thing we had in common). She stated her name was Roberta—more like Robert—and wanted to talk to "well hung" gentlemen. Again I pressed the number three, this time in a hurry.

I was expecting another freak, but this time the automated voice system told me I had a return message, and to press one to listen. As hurriedly as I'd pressed number three after hearing Roberta, I clicked on one.

"Hi Gary, this is Pauline. Thanks for your kind words. I love your accent, it sounds awesome. I'm part Skattish you know—on my father's side. Anyway, get back to me; let me know what you do for fun. Connect live if you'd like. I'd love to talk to you."

I tentatively pressed the number one key to connect live; a little nervous at the prospect of talking with a complete stranger, but relaxed a little as I giggled at the idea that this was exactly what a normal date would've been like for Stevie Wonder.

"Pauline?"

"Hey Gary, how are you?"

"Doing well, how about yourself?"

"Great; just hanging out surfing the line for a bit."

"Yeah, me too, but this is my first time on here."

"I do this all the time, I think it's awesome. I have literally a hundred friends on here now."

Alarm bells were already ringing in my head; surely someone that popular wouldn't be on here. I knew I would never classify someone as a friend if we had never met. An acquaintance perhaps, but a friend in my book was someone you *actually* hung out with.

"*Hundreds*," I said in a doubtful sounding tone, but it went straight over her head and she continued on.

"Yeah, it's great, and *so* much fun."

"That's cool; I'm just checking it out to see if I like it. What do you do for fun Pauline?"

"Just whatever, I really don't mind. I love the beach, drinking martini's, and driving around in my dad's BMW convertible—that is just *so* cool, especially here in Florida down on A1A. It's *so* awesome. The looks me and all my friends get from the guys walking around is *so* much fun."

I was actually losing the will to live. She was the complete opposite from what she'd sounded like in her ad and even on the message she left me. That was probably how she roped in guys to contact her. She spoke at one hundred miles an hour—one mph for every friend she had!—and hardly paused for breath. She was what me and my *actual* friends from back home termed a "whatever girl" in the way she would add about six R's to the end of the word—whateverrrrrr! I was half expecting her next line to be "and this one time," just like the movie American Pie.

"A BMW convertible, that sounds awesome!"

"It's *totally* awesome. My dad actually tells me he should just give the car to me as I drive it *way* more than he does," she boasted, chuckling like a school girl.

This girl had some serious issues, and I was beginning to feel like there was actually something mentally wrong with her. She was virtually a carbon copy of the stereotypical rich South Florida blonde bimbo, and I visualized a Paris Hilton look alike as she continued on her spoiled rant.

"One of my other friends on here is from Skatland as well. He is *really* awesome."

I pressed the number three key to disconnect the conversation. It may have been rude on my part, but I couldn't take her snobby bullshit any longer. I was positive if I'd handed her a world map and a pin, there would've been more likelihood of her sticking it in her eyeball than correctly pointing out exactly where "Skatland" was.

She was probably baffled by me disconnecting, but no doubt convinced herself I'd been on a cell phone and the call had accidentally dropped, and mentally penciled me in as friend one hundred and one!

This chat line reminded me of a story my friend Andy once told me. His older sister used to work for one of these sex lines back in England. She worked from home and had an ad in one of the local papers using the name "Sexy Sue" that showed a picture of a smoking hot young blonde in a bathing suit. She was inundated with calls from the lonely old perverted types looking for two minutes of fun talk with a saucy model type. She—real name Brenda—would have their toes curling as she described what she was wearing, or as it was usually communicated, what she wasn't wearing.

Brenda was actually a rather plump girl with dyed blonde hair. The extent of her sexy attire while she worked consisted of an oversized baggy t-shirt and her favorite pair of stained sweat pants. Guys would spend many expensive phone rate minutes on the call, believing she was naked and "playing" with herself, as they were "making her *so* horny." They weren't, and she never masturbated—on the phone line anyway.

The tools of her trade were a vibrator and a large orange with the top cut off. She would jam the buzzing toy in and out of the orange, creating a squelching noise while holding it to the telephone receiver. It must've been a convincing simulation, as she made a fortune from repeat callers who were convinced they had the power of bringing a hot young blonde to climax!

I marked down my experience with Pauline as being an anomaly and continued on.

My next conversation was with a woman named Maggie. She described herself as average looking, a little overweight, and in her early forties. She had a kind and caring tone to her voice, and although she was a little older than what I would usually date, I was only looking to chat and I admired the fact she was upfront about being partial to a carbohydrate or two, and not claiming to be a gorgeous super slim model.

"Maggie?"

"Hi there."

"How you doing? This is Gary."

"Nice to talk to you Gary. I love your accent. Where are you from?"

"Scotland."

"That's cool. What you up to this evening?"

"Not much, just hanging out at home and figured I'd give this chat thing a try. I'm pretty new to all this."

"Yeah, I'm fairly new to it as well. At least you sound remotely normal. You wouldn't believe some of the freaky guys I've bumped into on this line. They only seem to want someone to talk dirty to them or try and hook up and get into your pants."

She certainly was upfront. A quick hello and straight into telling me about men asking for sex!

"Well I'm just looking to chat for a bit. Not that I'm not into the whole sex thing. I mean I like sex, but I'm just looking for conversation. Sorry for babbling, I'm just a little nervous. You could never tell I'm a rookie at this!"

She let out a giggle and I knew she could virtually sense my inexperience and current vulnerability.

"So why did you come on the line Gary? What you looking for other than conversation?"

"I haven't really figured that out yet. I don't get out very much anymore and decided this might be a good way to talk to and maybe end up meeting someone nice."

"Well good luck with that. I hope the ladies on the line are nicer than the guys I've been bumping into. I don't mean to sound negative, but men generally seem to have a way of letting me down."

"Sounds like you've had a few bad experiences in your time."

"More than you wanna know about. I'm forty-three now and have lost count of the number of disappointments. Do you have a girlfriend?"

"Do you think I'd be doing this if I did?"

"You'd be surprised. A lot of them tell you they don't, but they do, and all they're looking for is a part-time fresh piece of ass."

"Do *you* have a boyfriend or husband?"

"I used to, but he turned out to be a real asshole. We were married for ten years. Turned out he was screwing my so called best friend behind my back for the last two of them. I thought something was going on. He started going out on his own a lot and got home at all hours of the night stinking of alcohol and shouting abuse at me. He even started slapping me around if I even questioned where he'd been."

That was *way* more information than I'd expected, and a rather frightening reply to my question—a simple "no" would've sufficed!

"Sorry to hear that. Sounds like you're better off without him."

"I know, I keep telling myself that, but deep down inside I still love him," she said, and I could almost see the tears filling up in her eyes.

"So what are *you* looking for on the chat line?" I replied, eagerly trying to change the direction our conversation was headed down.

I could've just disconnected the call like I'd done with Pauline, but deep down I was beginning to feel sorry for her, and didn't want to be categorized like all the other dead beats on the line she'd obviously encountered.

"Just someone nice to talk to; I'm still not over my ex and I have real trust issues now. I've been on a few dates since we split, but I just messed those up. They all went running for the hills and I'm sure they think I'm a jealous and emotionally unstable psycho."

"I'm sure they don't; sounds like they just weren't right for you."

"Thanks Gary, you're sweet. I just don't know what's happening inside my head anymore. I'm like a walking time bomb, and I'm almost afraid to be around people I don't know."

Her dates since the break-up probably did think she was a mental case, but I wasn't about to agree; sounded like she'd been through enough and obviously had a lot of issues, but I *could* relate to that, so decided to come clean and let her know she wasn't alone.

"I'm afraid to be around people as well."

"You are?"

"Maggie, I was diagnosed with arthritis when I was twenty-one. I've had a hip replacement already and my knee joints as so busted that I struggle to walk around unassisted at times, *and* I have a permanent limp. Shit, my shoulders, elbows, and ankles aren't much better."

"You're joking, right?"

"I wish I was, but I'm being straight up with you."

"You poor baby."

"Yeah, I know, but you just need to get on with things I suppose. I'm scared though. I see people looking at me strangely, wondering what's wrong with me and I hate the feeling it gives me inside. I used to be so active as well, and now I struggle to do the simplest of tasks, and it eats away at my sanity. It's just been easier for a while to separate myself from those around me and I've turned into a real social recluse, and it's not healthy. I figured I'd come on this line and at least try and kick-start some interaction without having anyone seeing my physical state."

It was weird talking about my problems with a stranger, but in an odd way I felt relieved.

Maggie and I chatted on for a while before we said goodbye, and I told her we could chat again on the line another time, even though I had no intention of coming back.

I lay on the sofa and pondered after I hung up the phone. The American women really dug the accent, so at least I had something going for me. The chat line wasn't really my thing, but it had been a real eye opener and made me realize there were a lot of mentally screwed up people out there—I *wasn't* alone. Maybe it was the norm as opposed to the extreme. I needed to pick myself up and get back out into the big bad world again. Perhaps there was hope and the future wasn't so bleak after all.

The Wonder Drug

I felt like I'd tried every form of prescription drug in the world of arthritis medication, but a change was about to occur. I'd seen my new rheumatologist a couple of times now, and she was seeing first hand that standard run of the mill treatments weren't helping.

"I'd like to try you on a new form of medication," said Dr. Kapila, my U.S. rheumatologist.

She was a wonderful little Indian woman, no more than five feet tall, jet black bobbed hair, and the most piercing blue eyes I'd ever seen; probably a result of their contrast against her light brown skin.

I'd only experienced a couple of rheumatologists in my time, but they were both fantastic caring people who knew just the right things to say at the appropriate time. They obviously sympathized with their patients and I assumed—rightly or wrongly—that all in their profession were likely of a similar persona.

"What type of new medication?"

"It's a fairly new drug on the market. It's been around for a couple years, but we don't have too much data on it compared to the medication you've been taking, as they've been around for a long time. The results we have been seeing with these new treatments though are extremely encouraging."

That was basically all I had to hear.

"Let's do it. I'll do *anything* if it might help."

She could tell from my tone of voice that I meant every word of it, and gave me a sad, almost motherly look. She felt bad for me, and knew I was desperate, and would reach out for any branch of hope that was thrown my way. She really was a sweetheart.

"OK, you have two options. One, you can administer the treatment yourself, or two, you can have it carried out in the outpatient department of the local hospital."

"It's not a pill?"

"No, it's given via injection. There's one that you would need to inject into your thigh every second day of the week. The hospital option would mean only one visit there for treatment every eight weeks. They would hook you up and deliver it over two hours intravenously."

"Option two please," I said with a smile, partly due to the potential new life-line and also from the fact I didn't want to stick a syringe into myself every other day.

She returned the smile, which basically informed me this was the common option selected by some of her other patients. Many people had a problem with needles, but I wasn't one of them; I'd been like a pin cushion over the years. Continual blood tests and steroid injections had grown me used to them.

Selecting the hospital option was more for convenience. One treatment every two months seemed far easier than making a schedule for myself, preparing the dose, and ultimately stabbing myself. I wasn't the most organized individual, so hospital it would be.

The drug was called Remicade (generic name Infliximab) and was a fairly new drug on the market used to treat autoimmune disorders such as arthritis and Crohn's disease.

I thoroughly researched its applications as well as success stories; which to my delight were plentiful. Its application and purpose was complex, but essentially it was a type of protein that recognizes, attaches to, and *blocks* the action of a substance in the body called tumor necrosis factor (TNF). TNF is made by blood cells in the body and can cause your immune system to attack *healthy* tissues in the body and cause inflammation and permanent damage to bones and cartilage; a process that had been affecting me for years, and was still in operation.

It was the morning of my first treatment. I enthusiastically drove my way to the hospital, not knowing what to expect, but joyful nevertheless. It was a typically warm day, but there was freshness in the air that was a pleasant change from the usual humid stuffiness. Maybe things in general were just beginning to change. Could this really be the drug that relieved me from this existence of hell?

I was delighted to see that a free valet service was available, an option I'd never seen before from any hospital in the UK. The British were so ass-backwards with that type of stuff. That was one of my major complaints about outpatient appointments back home. Hospital parking lots were generally packed, and I'd often have to endure a ten minute walk of pain and shame just to make it to the entrance. People muttering as they always did, no doubt feeling sorry for such a young man, struggling greatly with a look of agony on his washed out features. This wasn't an issue in the good ole US of A though.

The valet guy met me with a smile and was extremely patient as I slowly and stiffly removed myself from the driver's seat of my midnight blue V8 Ford Mustang and handed him the keys. I could tell he was wondering what was wrong with such a young guy. He was probably used to such a snail's pace from the thousands of geriatrics that frequented the place on a weekly basis, but not someone in their twenties. I could tell he liked the car though, so I made sure to take a mental note of the mileage in case he was thinking of taking it for a spin downtown to pick-up some chicks. It would've been the most action it had seen though since purchase and I thought maybe I could claim any score by default.

The car was the one thing that did make me happy. It was a little more expensive than I had planned to splash out on, but I figured it might inject some fun into my pathetic life. Some joked I was making up for manhood inadequacies, but even although I wasn't exactly hung like a Cheshire horse, I was really only making up for the fact I couldn't move around very fast.

I eventually made it to the registration office. The place was jammed with folks crammed in like farmyard animals. I gave my name to the hearing impaired elderly women at the desk, taking her four attempts before writing down what I assumed would be the correct spelling. Between her hearing and my accent, she was confused beyond belief. After her third attempt, I wished I'd just said Smith or Jones.

The waiting room was a sorry looking place, and further realization that I was one of many with problems. There weren't two people hanging the same way. There were wheelchairs, crutches, neck braces, the old and stooped, the young and bald.

I flicked through a copy of an entertainment magazine as I waited. It was out of date by around eighteen months. Even the pictures of George Clooney had him with a full head of brown hair. Today he was beginning to show some grey patches, but like Sean Connery, that only seemed to add to his handsome qualities.

I knew hospitals had a lot on their plates, but a quick run to the store by one of the many volunteers for some up to date reading material would've been a welcome addition.

Finally I was called to the registration desk by the same elderly lady.

"Barndon Wilkerson."

To no surprise she got it completely wrong, but it was close enough that I knew she meant me.

They wanted all sorts of information from me just so I could make it as far as the outpatient department. Driver's license, social security number, medical insurance card, do you have a living will, are you an organ donor, what's the square root of forty-nine? Here's my license, here's my social, insurance details on the bottom left, yes, no, seven. OK, slight exaggeration, but there *were* an endless number of questions. They even asked my current level of education. I was here for treatment of a disease, not interviewing for a position in the pediatrics department!

After ten minutes of interrogation, I limped my way to the nurses' station in outpatient surgery to give them my paperwork and no doubt hang around even longer in their waiting room. The paperwork I was carrying was as thick as J.K Rowling's latest novel. It was a complete waste of the environment, but almost heavy enough that if I carried it in my left hand it almost offset the limp caused by my right knee. Maybe a visit to Barnes and Noble would be on the agenda after I was done with the visit!

To my surprise, the head nurse, Linda, told me to go ahead and take a seat in the patient area. I almost needed a seat in order to get over the shock of not having to wait some more.

Linda pointed me towards an open plan area in the corner that looked like a cross between a treatment room and a medical storage area. In amongst the collection of wheelchairs and I.V. stands were four green leather lazyboy chairs in a square shaped formation. Three were occupied, so I sat down in the empty one and quickly realized why this one in particular remained vacant. I flicked the wooden handle on the side and popped up the foot support, only to find it wouldn't remain in an upward position under the weight of my legs, which was quite a feat considering my little bamboo sticks weighed no more than a couple of pool cues.

I was the youngest patient in the room by what seemed like fifty years. The gentleman closest to me appeared to be dead. He was hunched in his chair, chin resting against his chest, and so pale skinned it was verging on light blue. He was hooked up to a pump and was receiving a blood transfusion. I was just about ready to ask a nurse to check his pulse when suddenly he released a violent sneeze out of nowhere. He obviously had zero control of his ass muscles, as the force of the sneeze simultaneously triggered an enormous fart that echoed off the leather seat like an Austrian yodeling into a canyon.

In the next chair was a little plump Jewish lady who was acting as though she was being sponsored in a talkathon. She would *not* shut up. She didn't even pause for a breath as the old man's trumpeting butt went off. I think she was addressing the three of us in the room with her, yapping on about the outrageous house prices in the area and any other money related subject she could complain about. Nobody was really listening, but she kept going completely unfazed.

Patient number three was another elderly gentleman. He was wide awake, but staring into space in a trance-like fashion. He was receiving Remicade treatment as well, probably also for arthritis. I assumed he was still fairly functional though, as it appeared he'd managed to dress himself this morning. He was wearing a navy blue polo shirt and a pair of brown shorts, with the top of the waistband perched just below his nipples. The quality touch was the shin length white socks and open toe black sandals. If he *hadn't* dressed himself, the fashion police should've swung by his house and immediately arrested the guilty party.

"Mr. Wilkinson?"

I must've began to doze off, but opened my eyes to see an extremely attractive black nurse standing over me with Angelina Jolie type lips.

"Hi there."

"Hi Mr. Wilkinson, I'm Marcey, I'll be taking care of you this morning."

She had one of those low, sultry sounding voices that matched her beautiful appearance. Her body was tight also, and she was one of the few people I'd seen in my life who could pull off a pair of scrubs—so to speak. In fact I was convinced she would've still been a seven out of ten if she'd been clad in the old man socks and sandals attire.

"Hi Marcey, nice to meet you," I said, giving her a smile.

She returned the gesture, but her crystal looking teeth were *way* shinier than my nicotine tainted set.

"Call me Brandon, please."

"So Brandon, what's the Remicade for, arthritis or Crohn's disease?"

"Arthritis. I've got the joints of an eighty year old. No offense," I gestured to sandals boy, but he was still miles away in his own little world.

"This your first time receiving this medication?" she asked, preparing a syringe.

"Yeah, I'm a little Remicade virgin. I'm not quite sure what to expect. Hopefully it works better than the previous drugs I've been taking."

"I hope so. Hold still, this may sting a little," she replied, sinking the I.V needle into the pulsating vein on the back of my right hand.

I suppose it did sting a little, but it was barely noticeable in comparison to the pain I'd been living with for years.

"Aaaaaah," I yelped as the needle slipped into my skin."

"Oh, I'm sorry," said Marcey with a flinch and a look of concern.

"I'm just messing with you, it didn't hurt at all."

"You really are a brat aren't you?"

"I have my moments."

My confidence was sky high right now. It was weird, but it felt almost comfortable being here. I spent most of my life right now pretending I wasn't ill, but here everybody other than the staff *were* ill, so the penny finally dropped that I didn't have to kid myself here, and I was able to really let my hair down.

"I'll be back to check on you soon."

I was all hooked up to the clear bag of liquid medication, and I watched for a minute or so as it dripped down into the tube. I could feel it slip eerily into my system.

I sat back in my chair and gently drifted off.

"Wakey wakey, rise and shine."

I jumped to attention similar to a dream when you fall from a cliff.

"Hey Marcey; sorry I must've dozed off."

"Do you always snore so loudly?"

"Oh, you're kidding," I said, feeling the red warmth entering my embarrassed cheeks.

"Yes I am. See, two can play that game."

I liked her even more now; her personality aligning perfectly with her cute face and hot body.

"I'm done already?"

"Already, you've been sleeping for two hours!"

She wasn't kidding this time. My three geriatric companions were there no longer.

Marcey carefully removed the needle from me. The touch from her silky smooth hands was delightful, verging on a turn-on. It was the most physical female contact I'd had in a while, and it felt good, reminding me of nurse Jenny shaving me before my hip operation.

I said goodbye to her, throwing in a wink for good measure, and stiffly removed myself from the lazyboy. It had certainly lived up to its name during my visit.

I felt like crap; as stiff as I'd been in a long time. I convinced myself it was a result of falling asleep in a twisted position in the broken chair for so long.

I handed my ticket to the valet guy and waited patiently for his return, trying to stretch off my knees as much as possible while fighting through the pain.

He screeched to a halt in front of me. I was going to comment on the way he was driving my pristine car, but figured as long as the mileage was still intact I would let it slide, which turned out to be the case.

I drove wearily home, aching all over, and actually looking forward to awkwardly climbing into a hot bath. With a bit of luck the new medication would eventually give some relief. I wasn't expecting miracles, but I was expecting something to change. Hopefully there wasn't more heartbreak on the horizon.

Back on the Pies

Holy shit! This Remicade stuff *was* good. I had now been pain free for about a month. My mobility was still restricted as far as bending my knees and fully straightening my legs, and this would likely always be the case due to the irreversible cartilage damage the inflammation had caused, but I was OK with that. My lifestyle had changed anyway, and the prospect of not running again, playing soccer and other high activity level sports no longer bothered me. I could still hang with the best of them at pool and darts (pub games funnily enough!) and was now contemplating giving golf one more shot.

I was like a new man in terms of my appetite, and was wolfing down meat pies like it was a hotdog eating contest. It was difficult to say if it was just the new drug that was having this effect. It was obviously the major contributor, but mentally I was in heaven and content like back in the old days. I was a great believer that mood did contribute to overall well being and this combination was certainly working, and long may it continue.

For the first time I began paying close attention to my weight. I had been down to 106 lbs, which was verging on anorexic, but I had put on about ten pounds since my new treatment; eight of those probably due to the pies.

Told you so.

My imaginary friend was right. I was overcome with guilt as I recollected my time of weakness, vulnerability, and thoughts of taking my life. Things were certainly looking up.

I resisted temptation to weigh myself everyday, even though I wanted to. Change doesn't happen overnight, so I restricted it to a Sunday and Wednesday. I was rejuvenated by the gains I was achieving and was beginning to feel attractive again. I had a long way to go, but maybe the opposite sex would start to find me appealing once more and not just give me that look of feeling sorry for me. Either way, I had to get back out into the social world again and start trying. I began by shopping for some new "going out" clothes.

I hated the shopping malls at the weekend; they were crazy. The shear mention of the word "sale" had folks crawling out of the woodwork like a hungry pack of dogs. The hustle and bustle of it all annoyed me, and the rude South Florida attitudes drove me crazy. Whatever happened to common courtesy? People would bump into you as they slithered their way through the maze of fellow maniacs, never apologizing for doing so, and often would give you a stare like it was your fault for getting in the way of their next purchase.

My first port of call was the Versace store. It was a smart-looking shop, and you could almost smell the expensiveness in the air. The cost aspect didn't concern me; I had a high paying job and hadn't exactly been out socializing anywhere recently that would have depleted any funds, so my savings account was healthier than I'd been in a long time.

The interior of the store had a very minimalist look, so unlike many of the other outlet places that were crammed with rails and rails of clothing. Each stand had a very modern art décor feel to it, with twisting iron legs and shiny metal worktop surfaces, all clearly etched with the familiar Versace logo. Each shirt and pair of pants was folded immaculately, reminding me of the picture perfect stacks my mother used to create when folding the family laundry.

I was suspicious the management of the place was violating some of the anti-discrimination laws, or at least bending them to some degree, clearly to their advantage. Each of the assistants would've been at home modeling for any fashion catalogue, decked out in their designer gear and had jaw-dropping features that only added to the appeal of the place. Surely some unattractive people must have submitted a job application—including mandatory photograph—in the past, but were conveniently sent a rejection letter "sympathizing" that they'd been unsuccessful on this occasion.

"Can I help you sir?" inquired a striking tall female with short black layered looking hair, with a sliver of bright pink running through it.

She could've helped me all right; I hadn't been laid in a while, but I was certain that the thoughts flooding my mind weren't being reciprocated.

"Just looking around, but I'll be sure to let you know if I need any help".

"My name's Mandy."

"Nice to meet you Mandy, I'll give you a shout if I need you."

She turned and made her way back to the counter; her buttocks were tight and filled every inch of her short black miniskirt. It was as though they were almost talking to me; "spank me Brandon, spank me." I really had to get some action, and quickly, I was becoming delusional! She had on knee length black boots as well, a real favorite of mine, and her overall look was almost punkish—it was a real turn on.

The owners of the shop were pure genius. I hadn't even inspected any of their clothing items yet, but I'd already decided I was going to buy something, just because I wanted some further interaction with the wonderful Mandy and her tight ass—it was almost pathetic, but I was sure I wasn't the first to fall into their little trap, and certainly wouldn't be the last.

A pair of slick-looking black jeans with a thin white pinstripe caught my eye. They had them in my petite size as well, which was always a concern when I entered a store. I held them up to my legs as I stared into the trendy oval shaped mirror—they were perfect. A quick glance at the price tag altered my selection process. Three hundred dollars! I wasn't concerned so much with the expense as I was about being clearly ripped off. They were fantastic looking, but the thickness of the material gave the impression you could've spat through them. Needless to say they were returned to their original location in the blink of an eye, and I headed towards the t-shirt section.

The t-shirts were hot-looking, much like the luscious Mandy, and even although they were also a little pricey, I could at least get half a dozen of them for the same cost as the pinstripe jeans.

I gave Mandy a glance and she caught my eye as I held up a few shirts.

"Wanna try them on?" she asked with a flirtatious grin.

This girl was born to sell, and I could almost see the commission dollars flash in her eyes already.

"Absolutely, they're really smart-looking."

"The red one will go really well with your skin tone."

Boy, she was *good*. The red shirt would've been as well to walk its ass to the register right now and fall into one of their fancy store bags.

I smiled and followed in the direction of the changing rooms. The rhythmical movement of her tight butt cheeks was mesmerizing; her catwalk style prance only enhancing the wiggle. I was almost glad I wasn't trying on the pants, as it would've required some gymnastic type moves to get the current pair off such was the ever growing swelling taking place in my groin.

"I'll be right out here if you need anything."

"Thanks Mandy," I said, pulling back the silky curtain.

The curtain was like a two way mirror. I wasn't able to see into any of the other occupied rooms, but from inside I was able to see out through the material; I'd never encountered anything like it before. Most other places just had a plain old wooden door, but I guess that wasn't suave enough for Versace.

Like she'd stated, Mandy was indeed right outside, and I found myself day-dreaming all over again as my eyes traced the exterior of her entire body. I was sure her breasts were a pair of stick-ons—a Scottish phrase for having implants—but that wouldn't have stopped me mauling them given half a chance, even though I definitely preferred the feel of the "au naturale" versions.

"How you getting on in there?" said Mandy, almost causing me to shriek as I quickly awakened from my fantasy.

"Great, you were right about the red one, looks great," I lied, scrambling to get my shirt off.

"Give us a look then."

Shit, I had to work fast, but was eager to show her and gauge the reaction.

"Give me a second."

I pulled back the curtain and her intense green eyes roamed across my shoulders, chest and stomach.

She rolled her R's resembling a cat like purr.

"Rrrrrrr."

She was probably just pushing for a sale, but for the first time in ages I really had the feeling of being attractive again.

"You took the words right out of my mouth," I said with a wink. "I said the exact same thing to myself as I stared into the mirror in there!"

She laughed loudly. My confidence was growing like my earlier erection and I was ready to take on the world again.

"I'll just take them all; they're the same size anyway."

"Sure you don't want to try on the others?"

"Positive, I'm in a bit of a rush anyway, got a lunch date," I exclaimed rather smugly, even though it was complete fiction.

"Well you'll be looking even better for her with your new clothes."

"Yeah, I think you might be right."

I gave Mandy a smile and a wave as I left the store. I was feeling great, but not good enough to ask her out for dinner or anything. Don't run before you can walk was my motto, but maybe I would get up the courage if I visited the place again and she was around. I wanted to leave her thinking I was a bit of a player, meeting a hot chick for lunch and perhaps had another one on the go for the evening shift; keep her on her toes. It couldn't have been further from the truth, but she didn't know that.

Me, Myself and I

There was no doubt I now resembled more of my former self. The pain was gone, and even although my flexibility wasn't great, life was good again. An inner scar had been created though that was an entirely different challenge to resolve.

Years of mental trauma had essentially turned me into a "closed shop," and my lack of ability to express myself emotionally to those close to me had become ingrained. I hated talking about the past as it created nightmares of times I wanted to remain behind lock and key. Any time they invaded my fragile mind they would have a negative impact on my mood.

Intimate relationships were a worry. Not only had I been hurt before, but times with women during my illness had me pushing them away rather than embracing them into my world of emotional turmoil. It had become my way, almost cast in stone, and like any major change, this one would be a tough one to break free from.

The prospect of a new relationship terrified me, but I was going to have to deal with such situations at some point. I figured I could lie and refuse to disclose my condition, but the guilt factor ruled that out as a possible option. I was scared to fall in love again. If my disease deteriorated again, which was always a possibility, I still didn't want to burden anyone with sharing my pain and anguish. In addition, I wasn't prepared for the heartache should anyone break-off our relationship. Even if it was genuinely for any reason other than my condition, part of me would always wonder if that was really the truth. It was easier to avoid these encounters altogether, but I had to try and break free from this line of thinking.

One thing was for sure; the type of woman I *could* become involved with had become restricted to certain parameters. I couldn't find myself with someone who was the active, outdoors type, who enjoyed high intensity sports on the weekend like Liz back in the UK. That would gradually fizzle out due to us not having much in common. That would've been true, but deep down the root cause would've been my physical limitations. It wasn't that I didn't want to have such things in common, more that I couldn't.

I needed a cute, bubbly character who enjoyed social interaction in a bar setting. Someone who liked to shoot a game of pool or darts; something I could still participate in.

My plan was in place. As much as I hated the restrictions, I had to deal with them in a positive manner and move forward with my life.

Haven't I Seen You Somewhere Before?

I felt I'd been awakened from a five year coma, rejuvenated and ready to find myself again. This was a revelation, finally realizing there *was* hope. The tunnel had been a long and excruciating one, but the light was clearly in view, beaming bright, with a warm comforting glow to it. I was careful not to get ahead of myself, as day turns into night, and the light may slowly change back to a dark, cold sky. I would take it one day at a time and start to live again. My confidence had reached new heights and the world no longer appeared as the big bad place it had previously become.

It was Friday, and the work day sailed by. My mood was upbeat as I merrily chatted with my colleagues, many asking if I "was on something." I was, life, and it was providing me with a high better than any illegal narcotic. I hardly performed a stroke of work the entire day. There was nothing urgent on my plate that couldn't wait until Monday morning. I was focused on the now, and eagerly anticipating a night of fun.

I arrived in a taxi at Declan's place around nine thirty, giving the Indian driver a fabulous tip and bringing a beaming smile to his face that had previously been the definition of miserable since I climbed into his body odor tainted cab. My mood was electric and I wanted to share the joy.

As usual, Declan wasn't even close to being ready, which I'd already anticipated as I sent Ravi on his merry way.

"Alright horse box," said Dec, greeting me at the door in only a pair of boxer shorts. The phrase "horse box" was an Irish term that even to this day I have no idea of its origin. Pick a word to substitute—mate, chief, buddy, it was all the same.

"Not bad mate, ready for a few cold ones, that's for sure."

"Gimme fifteen minutes and I'll be ready to roll. I'm right in the mood for a few scoops myself."

I took a seat in the living room as Dec disappeared off to freshen up and prepare for a drunken night, hoping it ended with some one on one with a fine young American lass.

His apartment was the ultimate definition of a bachelor pad. A photograph of his front room would've been way more descriptive than any words defining the phrase. Dirty dishes cluttered the sink of the open plan kitchen, three empty pizza boxes were spread out over the counter tops like strategically placed ornaments, and the dishwasher appeared to glisten like new—a direct result of a lack of use.

I grabbed the TV remote and sat slouched on the end of his black leather three seat sofa, one of the few sensible purchases that any woman may have been proud of him for. Adjacent to the couch was a white plastic single seat chair, the outdoor type you often find around swimming pools. I think he'd picked it up for eight dollars from Home Depot, the time he'd gone for screws with the purpose of putting up a shelf. The screws were still in their unopened pack, lying beside one of the pizza boxes. The TV was perched on top of the box it had been delivered in, and he hadn't even attempted to disguise it as a table by covering it with a sheet, drape or any form of material that would hide the word "Panasonic" in huge black lettering. The walls were as bare as a baby's bottom, not a picture or framed photograph to be found. The only interruption to the plain, smooth white surfaces was a small hole near the bedroom door; the result of an off center hit from chipping golf balls on a boring midweek night.

"Clan you clall a clab?" came the cry from the bathroom.

Why he couldn't remove the toothbrush from his mouth for a second was beyond me, but I searched around for the portable phone to put in another call to Ravi's taxi firm. Not to my surprise the receiver was nowhere to be seen. I rummaged behind the sofa cushions and finally found the phone, after pocketing seventy-five cents in spare change and an apple flavored Jolly Rancher.

"OK, let's get this show on the road," said Dec, appearing like a transformed character from the steamy bathroom, just like the hit TV show Stars in Your Eyes.

He was certainly out to impress, and I felt a little underdressed in my blue 501's and polo shirt. He was wearing a pressed pair of beige trousers and a smart black shirt with silver buttons and the words "Hugo Boss" hugging his left nipple area like a small fashionable name tag. If only he took as much pride with his apartment!

We hung around outside the complex for only a few minutes before seeing the familiar yellow light on top of the car pulling into the street. A bright white set of teeth were visible through the windshield, it was Ravi again, no doubt anticipating another hefty tip as he recognized my presence.

"Christ, it smells like something died in here!" exclaimed Dec, pulling a face like he'd just dropped an egg-tainted fart.

I was going to warn him before hand, but figured he would be as politically correct in his vocal expression as an obnoxious drunk realizing he'd just pissed himself. The look on Ravi's face was priceless as his smile turned upside down and he attempted to discreetly sniff his festering armpit.

We made our way speedily in the direction of TGI Fridays, which was generally packed—ironically enough—on a Friday evening. The female bartenders were hot, and generously intermingled with a fair share of available female customers; one of the main purposes of our visit. Like any bad smell, the aroma from Ravi's lively armpits grew on our nostrils, and had all but disappeared by the time we reached the bright red and white striped sign of our destination.

The music pulsed at a medium volume as the few remaining diners tackled their over indulgent chocolate desserts. The beats progressed in loudness as the food lovers dispersed, leaving those purely pursuing alcohol to continue the party.

We found two remaining seats at the bar and relaxed into them as though we'd just completed a physically draining marathon run.

"What can I do for you gentlemen this evening?" asked Tanya the barmaid, subconsciously sticking her chest out in our direction.

"More than you could probably imagine," I said with a wink. "But we'll make do with two Sam Adams, for now anyway."

Dec laughed as Tanya returned a smile, perhaps flattered with the obvious advance, but maybe a result of realizing she was tending on two desperate suckers who'd be lining her pockets with money by the end of the evening if she maintained the flirtatious exchanges.

The beers were going down a treat as we talked about work, sports, and how great breasts were, our conversation occasionally interrupted as we paused and gazed like a couple of sex starved imbeciles each time a reasonably hot girl walked by in the direction of the bathroom. Each time we wondered if they were going number one or number two. This determination turned into a game; length of time to return being the factor built into our decision making process. We really were a couple of pigs, and it was a wonder how we'd ever managed to score, never mind hold down any form of relationship. Perhaps that was the reason we were currently single.

Our delusional playing around was abruptly interrupted as a group of five girls entered the bar, loudly giggling, and obviously not the first bar they'd visited this evening. They were a mixed-looking bunch as often groups of women were; two extremely attractive ones, two that were definitely worth a roll in the sack in about three beers time, and one who couldn't have enticed the Elephant Man from a burning house.

I always felt a little bad for the ugly one of any group of ladies. They obviously knew the others were a few leagues higher in the looks department, but perhaps they were comforted by the fact they would at least be exposed to some male attention as a result of their more attractive buddies.

Guys were total dogs anyway—Dec and myself aware we were just part of the norm and not a couple of perverted freaks. If five guys were interacting with this group of gals, one of them would've likely taken one for the team; the concept being that some loving is better than none at all and still a step higher up the ladder than palm and her five sisters.

The girls grabbed one of the available wooden high top tables about ten feet or so from the bar, giving us a perfect view of them and full exposure to their antics and enthusiastic conversation. There were three brunettes, one with jet black hair, and the lone ugly blonde. I was instantly attracted to one of the brunettes. She was facing in my direction and the gleam from her smile was giving me a warm feeling inside—I only wished it had been aimed at me. Her face was maybe the most beautiful sight I'd ever encountered. It was flawless; seemingly blemish free, and significantly tanned, giving her an almost Mediterranean flavor. Her dark brown eyes were like a couple of sparkling exotic jewels, and the shiny lip gloss she was wearing added a juiciness to her full lips that made me want to immediately feel them pressed against mine.

Their initial cheerful personas were deteriorating though as they looked around the bar, presumably for a waitress so they could continue their evening of drinking. The place was becoming packed though, and nobody was around to relieve them of their thirst. To my delight, my dream girl approached the bar area adjacent to Dec and myself. She timidly squeezed her way in between two middle-aged gentlemen and a younger couple, and proceeded to order drinks. Wow, they were all beer drinkers, a slightly uncommon event for a group of females, but a sure sign they were partial to more than one or two.

Dec gave me a nudge in the side.

"Sweet," he said.

"Unbelievable," was all I could muster as a reply.

I was almost in a trance as she handed over money to Tanya. I had to think fast. Opportunities like these didn't present themselves everyday, so I had to say something, preferably with some original wit to it.

"Excuse me," I said, getting her attention.

My heart pounded as her gaze met mine and my mind went blank.

"Haven't I seen you somewhere before?" Great line! It had about as much original wit to it as the winner of the 'Mr. Lack of Original Wit' contest.

She gave me a puzzled look before a smirk appeared on her glorious features.

"Yes, I think we have. That's why I don't go there anymore!"

She smiled before turning around and skillfully carried the five bottles of cold beer back to her awaiting audience, no doubt to detail her brief encounter with some slime bag with the worst chat up line since records began!

"I think you might be in there!" exclaimed Dec, laughing almost uncontrollably.

"I'm an idiot. Haven't I seen you somewhere before? What kind of bullshit line was that?" I said, letting my forehead fall into the palms of my hands.

"A bad one."

"No shit Sherlock."

"Think they're talking about you now," said Dec, cheesy grin still on his face.

I looked over in horror as five giggling versions of Dec stared back at me. As my eyes met their table, the laughter intensified and I felt my cheeks reddening more with every chuckle they made.

"I'm not giving up on that one yet. One thing I'm not is a quitter."

"Yeah, but sometimes it's better to quit while you're ahead—or behind in your case."

"Hey, at least she was smiling."

"Maybe if you bump into her again one day you can ask her the same question. She'll probably say, yeah, you're the douche bag with the fantastic chat up lines!"

He had a point, but I wasn't about to admit defeat just yet. My confidence was soaring in my life right now, even in light of the more than unsuccessful first impression.

We finished off a few more cold dark beers, intermittently watching a Miami Heat and Los Angeles Lakers basketball game on the TV screen hovering over the bar.

"Looks like they're ready for another round," said Dec, pointing me in the direction of the girls table.

Tanya was right beside us topping up a soda refill with the shower head pump.

"Tanya, the next round for the girls over there is on me," I said, gesturing in the direction of the ladies as they debated who was going to be the unlucky one making the venture to the bar.

Hopefully their debate was not to see who drew the short straw and have to deal with the two foreign idiots sitting there.

One of the friends made her way up, squeezing her way timidly next to the loving young couple. She ordered from Tanya, who quickly proceeded to open the caps on the five bottles and inform the cute brunette that they were on me.

"Thanks," she said, simulating the universal sign with her bottle that meant "cheers" from where I was from.

"You're welcome. Tell your friend I apologize for the pathetic chat up line. I do think she is cute though."

"You didn't do too badly, she's been talking about you ever since she came back from the bar," she replied, and instantly took the bottles and made her way back to their table.

She was quick on the retreat, much to my dismay. I'd been hoping to interrogate her further after her positive comment, but I was too late. Things were looking up though.

Dec looked at me with a quick shrug of his eyebrows.

"Told you mate, you've either got it or you haven't and I certainly don't fall into the latter," was my response, even although I was genuinely surprised with what just occurred. I had actually thought I'd screwed things up completely and should be looking around for new prey if I was hoping for a score this evening.

"Fair play to you mate, I thought you had blown it."

"To be honest with you chief, I thought I had as well. Anyway, let's bump our heads together and figure out a strategy. If she's been talking about me constantly it means she might be interested. If that's the case you've got four to choose from. OK, three if we don't include Quasi."

"At this moment in time mate, Quasi is getting cuter by the mouthful anyway. Right now I'd probably shove it in a hairy donut, so don't worry about it."

"You really are a dog, but I kinda feel the same way right now. I haven't had the touch of a good woman for way too long. The hand holding hospital incident really doesn't count."

"Whatever you wanna do mate."

"Well we could go over there after this beer and give them a bit of the old Irish and Scottish charm, but if that chick was having a laugh we could completely bomb, turn around and find that someone had pinched our seats, then we're completely back to square one without anywhere to sit."

"Good point chief. I've been kinda getting the eye from our Tanya lass anyway, so the last thing I want is to potentially screw up both options right now."

"OK, it's a done deal. We wait till they come back to the bar, ask if they'd like some company. If they say no we cut our losses, you hit on Tanya and I pick another target for the night. Sound like a plan?"

"Works for me mate."

We ordered up another couple of Sam Adam's and continued on our conversation, including our bathroom number guessing game. I kept one eye on the girls, and the more I watched, the more I believed the friend who'd given us the down low on the situation. My girl would often give me a look, a brief one, but a look nevertheless. Even her friends would look up now and again. Hopefully at least one of them was deciding on who was leaving with Dec.

They may have been beer drinkers, but they were a hell of a lot slower in getting them down the hatch than me and the Dec boy. It seemed like an eternity before they were ready for another. We'd already chugged another two before the girls approached again.

Miss Modo got up from her seat and made her approach, much to the delight of both of us. It was *way* easier to talk to an average-looking girl than a really hot one. I wasn't sure why that should be the case, but probably because there was a universal belief that they were more receptive to strange boys talking to them, as it was more of a rarity rather than the norm for her more facially gifted friends.

She made her way clumsily towards the beer pumps, her ample hips fiercely nudging a few strangers as she *attempted* to elegantly tip-toe her way past unnoticed.

Surprisingly enough—much against my first belief—she looked a little better up close than from a distance; not much, but she'd advanced to a four out of ten. If she'd actually taken the time to apply some make-up and invest in a stylish haircut, she may even have advanced another notch. Two months at the gym would also have helped, but regardless of the additional effort, she would've topped out at a six, which was a perfectly acceptable number under intoxicated circumstances.

I took a double take after those thoughts. Who the hell was I to judge the looks of anybody? Don't get me wrong, I'd put on about ten pounds in weight since the beginning of my treatment, but I wasn't exactly model material myself and should feel lucky that her gorgeous friend was even showing the slightest interest in me.

The plan was laid. She was going to order their drinks, we'd wait until she was paying and then approach the subject of joining them at their table; a plan that went south in a hurry.

"So you are the guys who've been checking us out all night," came the completely unexpected words from her.

We were tongue-tied, caught off guard, feet stuck firmly in our oversized mouths.

"We may have looked over a couple of times," said Dec to the rescue.

I was lost for words and hadn't expected a peep from the girl.

"I might not be the finest diamond in the box of rocks, but I could tell you were giving us the eye. Not necessarily me, as it generally never is, but I can still tell you guys got it bad."

Her blatant confidence was unbelievable, but at the same time was rocketing her point accumulation towards the two friends in the median scoring zone.

"OK you got me. I really admire your honesty. There's no beating about the bush with you is there? What's your name?" inquired Dec.

"I'm Debbie. And yeah, there's no bush beating with me, I'm purely heterosexual."

She might not have been the most physically attractive female in the world, but what she lacked in looks, she certainly made up for in personality. Dec was sitting there, mouth open, and I got the feeling he was accelerating her up the scale at a rapid rate of knots.

"You're quite the little fire cracker," said Dec, finally closing his mouth and uttering a few words.

"By the way, not that you probably care, but I've been checking *you* out since *I've* been here," she directed at Dec as she skillfully grabbed the five beers in her hands and made her way back to the table.

We were both left sitting there open-mouthed again. Pausing halfway to her table Debbie turned around.

"Do you guys need more of an open invitation to join us or what?"

We looked at each other briefly and swiftly grabbed our drinks.

The conversation was flowing, Dec sandwiched between Debbie and Victoria, the hottest looking one—in my opinion—besides Teri. Teri was the object of my desires and we were involved in a heated debate about whether the Scottish accent was more attractive than the Irish one. I was ready to consult Dec on this one, but figured as he was Irish born and bred he would've quickly sided with

Teri. I wasn't convinced whether she was genuinely in favor of Ireland or whether she was doing everything in her power to mess with me.

"We've got Sean Connery, who does Ireland have?"

"Well there's Liam Neeson for starters and that Michael Flatley from River-dance is pretty hot."

"Michael Flatley! I've never even heard that guy talk, so I doubt you have. He might be good with his legs but there's no way you can back up his conversation skills. He's probably as dull as the Irish sky. Anyway, he's not completely Irish. His parents were, but I think he was born in Chicago or something."

"He's still sexy. Besides, all Sean does is pronounce his S's in a weird way."

"Oh do you think sho pooshy," I replied, giving her my best impersonation.

"Well now you put it like that, perhaps we can call it a draw and move on."

"Well thank you Mish Money Penny."

She giggled at that one and gave me a prolonged stare that had me weak at the knees and thankful that I was sitting down.

"I think it's time we were getting out of here," said Victoria, apparently bringing an abrupt end to the party.

"I think I'm going to hang around for another drink," said Debbie, looking lustfully into Dec's eyes, much to his excitement.

"I think I should stay and chaperone Debbie," said Teri, flashing a not so discrete wink towards Victoria.

It was music to my ears, and Declan. Even through his drunken state he was giving me a sneaky thumbs up signal.

The three friends swigged down the remains of their drinks and headed on their way. The other two of them, Rachael and Pamela, who'd barely said a word to us all night, left in the same way, obviously not happy with our arrival or the fact some of their friends were sticking around for more. I got it in my head that they were annoyed that Debbie and Teri had landed a couple of winners, but deep down I knew that was nonsense.

I approached the bar for a final round of drinks, glad I had my back to them all, as I had a huge smile on my face. What a result. I could still hardly believe it, particularly the fact she genuinely seemed to like me.

"Two Sam Adams and two Miller Lites please Tanya."

"Looks like someone might be getting lucky tonight," she said with a smirk.

"Yes, I think she probably will be," I replied smugly.

"I didn't mean her."

"I know you didn't, but I just like being a smart-ass."

I carefully carried the four bottles back to the table, weaving my way through the traffic of fellow drinkers. I was really starting to feel drunk, so was glad this was the last one of the evening. I wasn't quite sure what was going to materialize after we left the bar, but didn't want to get too plastered in case I "got lucky" as Tanya so eloquently put it, and run the risk of falling asleep before anything physical kicked off.

"So where do you live, Dec?" said Debbie.

"Only about a mile north of here on Pine Island Road."

"Really. I'm only about another three miles north of that. Would you mind if I shared a cab with you on the way home?"

Our Debbie certainly wasn't shy. She would've been as well saying "do you mind if I come home with you and we can participate in a horizontal workout?"

"Not at all. We can go now if you'd like?"

"Sounds good to me," said the eager Debbie, swallowing down half a beer in one go.

Dec gulped the remainder of his drink down at a rapid rate of knots, and for a moment I thought the entire bottle was going to disappear down his throat, such was the urgency to get back to his bedroom.

"Alright guys, we'll catch you later. Teri, it was great to meet you. Chief, I'll give you a call tomorrow.

Debbie said a quick goodbye and they almost jogged to the exit.

"Holy crap, there was no messing around with those two," I said, almost in disbelief.

"Yeah, Debbie isn't really known for her tact."

"Well, I'd share a taxi home with you, but unlike those two I live in the complete opposite direction from you Teri."

"Well you could come back to mine for a cup of coffee if you'd like."

"That would be nice, but I'm not really in the mood for a coffee."

"Neither am I, but I'm sure we'll think of something."

The Grand Slam

The sun was up as we opened the front door of her apartment and I kissed Teri goodbye on the doorstep, having made sure to brush my teeth prior to doing so. I hoped I'd used her toothbrush, but there were three to choose from in the bathroom, so there was around a 66% chance it was one of the roommates; the two sour-faced broads from the previous night, so regardless I wasn't concerned, and even managed a giggle.

We kissed again as the yellow cab pulled up in front of the apartment block.

"I had a really nice time last night. I hope we can get together again," I said, really staring deeply into her beautiful brown eyes.

She looked just as good in the morning. Her make-up was removed and she had her hair pulled back in a ponytail, but surprisingly it didn't do her any injustice, which was a rarity, as often you could wake-up with a woman and feel like inquiring where the hot chick was that you went home with the previous evening.

"Call me later; maybe we can go see a movie tonight or something."

"I'd really like that," I replied, glad in the fact she seemed as interested in me as I was in her.

I felt I looked like ass as well; same clothes as the night before, including underwear, no time for a shower, and I had a serious dose of bed head that no amount of water or hair gel could completely flatten.

We shared another quick smooch before I climbed into the fusty smelling taxi.

It was just after ten, so I called Dec on my cell phone as the cab belted its way along—engine warning light on—towards my lonely apartment.

"How you doing chief?" I said to Dec in a raised voice as the foreign driver bellowed into his radio in Arabic or something.

"Empty," was his only word.

"I assume you got lucky then. Either that or you went home alone and gave your wrist a good workout."

"Well I wasn't alone, and the only exercise my wrist was doing was on her. She was an animal. We just did it again about an hour ago. My manhood is glowing in the dark this morning. Listen, she's gone already, meet me at Denny's and I'll buy you a Grand Slam."

"No worries. I'm on my way. I'll be there in about ten minutes or so."

Denny's was its typical Saturday morning state—filled to the rafters with people too lazy to cook their own breakfast, and there was an ever-growing waiting list of families to be seated, becoming more and more impatient as every minute passed.

Dec and I were seated fairly quickly though as it was just the two of us. It was a relief to me as the little impatient rug-rats running about in the lobby had been continually running into my legs. I was feeling good and didn't want any preventable knock sending me back into pain again.

Our elderly waitress, Doris, filled our coffee mugs to the brim as we thumbed our way through the menu. I really was feeling great this morning; not an ache to be found, and my frame of mind was at an all time high as I had a permanent picture of Teri's beautiful face etched in my brain.

"So, Debbie was a bit of a handful then."

"A couple of good handfuls," he said, simulating a pair of breasts with his cupped hands. "Nothing I couldn't handle, so to speak."

"You going to see her again?"

"Hell no. I'm sure she's feeling the same. It was as though I was only serving one purpose for her last night and again this morning. As soon as we were done she put her clothes on, called a taxi, and was on her way without any of the BS about giving her a call or any emotional attachment at all for that matter. Cool girl, I wish more of them worked that way. It would save me a fortune on phone calls and dinner dates. How did it go with you and Teri?"

"Fantastic. She really is a sweetheart."

"You gonna see her again?"

"Hopefully tonight."

"It must've been good."

"It was, but there's more to it than that. I really felt like there was a strong connection."

Doris jotted down the details for our super-sized breakfasts and topped up the coffee, talking to us about where our accents were from, but all I could think about was Teri and seeing her again tonight.

An Early Confession

I eagerly drove my Ford Mustang in the direction of Teri's place; the roar of the V8 engine aligned with my inner feeling of excitement.

I said I'd be over around seven thirty, and for once in my life it looked like I was going to be on time for a date.

It was time to be a man on this occasion and not shy away from my illness and pretend it didn't exist. No, this time the cards would be immediately laid on the table, no messing around. It would be a little easier anyway. For one, we'd just met, and two, I was looking and feeling better, so it wasn't like evidence of a crippled young man was there for all to see. I was still a little on the skinny side, but that was on the increase by the pie.

I parked the car in the dimly lit lot outside her place, fortunate enough to find an empty spot directly under the only tall light pole. I loved my car and wanted to use every deterrent I could to prevent a possible break-in. I beeped the alarm and took a few deep breaths as I made my way to the front door, giving it a rhythmical knock with four quick ones, a very brief pause, then two more in swift succession. I hoped Teri would be the one to respond instead of one of her sour-faced roommates who would've no doubt made me feel as welcome as a fart in an elevator.

"Hey there," she said, beaming smile and hair restored to its elegance of the previous night.

"Great to see you again," I replied, giving her a tight hug and quick peck on her sweet lips.

"Well we have the place to ourselves, so we can either go out to a movie or watch one here."

"A cozy night in sounds good to me. To be honest I'm still feeling a little rough from the alcohol last night."

"I was hoping you'd say that. I've been a little under the weather today myself."

We snuggled up as one on the soft sofa as Ocean's Eleven played on the large TV screen set inside the pine wood entertainment unit. I tried to pay as much attention to the movie as possible, but the fresh aroma of her sexy perfume was a serious distraction.

No sooner had Clooney, Pitt, Damon and the other eight pulled off the heist and the credits rolled, I decided it was time.

"Listen Teri, there's something I wanna tell you."

"Don't tell me you used to be a woman," she said with a serious look, followed by a cheesy grin and some laughter.

She had a superb personality. Her wit was as sharp as a razor, and a quality as rare as a slice of beef that never made it to the grill.

"Telling you I was a woman would be easier than this!"

That certainly got her attention.

"Seriously though, I don't have a vagina but I do have an incurable disease."

"WHAT!"

Her face went ghost white and my delivery was *way* harsher sounding than I had intended, but it got her to be quiet *real* quick. I was sure she was envisioning HIV or Herpes, or had a few others driving erratically through her mind, so I had to work fast.

"Calm down, it's not what you think. It's nothing of a sexual nature."

"Go on."

"I've got arthritis. You probably haven't noticed or can't tell right now, but I do. I've had it for a few years now but it seems to be in remission at the moment."

"And you're telling me this why?"

"Well I like you and want to be open with you."

"Oh, you like me do you. I was hoping I'd hear you say that."

"I'm sure I gave away that fact very clearly already."

"I suppose, but I can never tell at times. Anyway, I noticed you had a slight limp, but I figured you just had a sore leg or something. I didn't see the point in bringing it up."

I did still have a slight limp. I was pain free, but years of bad posture and the remaining fact that my joints were still damaged had those mechanical motions ingrained.

"Well as I said, I just wanted to be upfront with you."

"Brandon, I'm not looking for some chiseled hunk with a body you can break rocks off and participates in the Florida track and field team. I'm a little less pretentious than that! Mental stimulation is more important to me, and you certainly do a good job at that. Anyway, I've not been without a few physical issues myself."

"How do you mean?"

"I've already had three back surgeries. I had a severely herniated disc in my spine that was impacting my sciatic nerve root. It is still painful at times when I do too much. I can't participate in any high intensity sports or lift anything heavy, as that would almost cripple *me*," she said, pulling up the back of her shirt to expose about a four inch vertical scar.

We'd already been intimate, but the room had been dark at the time, so I hadn't noticed, just like she hadn't noticed my hip scar.

"I'm sorry to hear that."

"Well if that bothers you then maybe we don't take this any further," she said with a frown.

"Don't be ridiculous."

"I know I'm being ridiculous; I'm just trying to make a point. I *really* don't care about your condition. Good guys are hard to find, and you're certainly a good one. Plus you've got that sexy Sean Connery thing going on."

"Yesh, you make an exshellent point Pooshy," I replied, becoming smugger by the second.

"Now shtop you're nonshensh Mishter Wilkinshon and give me a kish."

She was hilarious. We embraced with a magnetic-like passion. Her acceptance of me for who I was filled me with the type of excitement I hadn't felt in a long long time.

I was genuinely sorry that she'd had serious back problems, but a slight selfish component inside me was comfortable with it. She could understand pain, surgery recovery, temporary lapses, and the fact I'd never be Mr. Active.

This *was* the beginning of a beautiful thing.

It's a Wonderful Life

It had been over six weeks since my first Remicade treatment and I was *still* essentially pain free. I was on cloud nine right now. Nothing ached other than the occasional twinge, and things between Teri and I were only flourishing.

It was like we'd know each other for many years, childhood sweethearts almost. She laughed at my corny jokes, had deep and meaningful conversations about real world issues such as global warming, third world poverty, and other cerebral topics such as domestic healthcare problems. Those subjects weren't everyone's idea of a good time, but it was great to be with someone where intellectual chit-chat was an option if you wanted it to be. Physical stimulation is a must, but can only carry a relationship so far. If there was such a phenomenon, mental orgasm was now an option for me; a combination not found in the repertoire of many couples these days, especially if current divorce rates were anything to go by.

Although she'd been in Florida for a while, Teri was from the Upper Peninsula of Michigan; almost Canada if you were looking at an atlas. She had that northern mentality; down to earth, actually appreciated sarcasm, and could sup down a beer like a Scottish lass. Combined with the fact she was smoking hot made her the ultimate package. Tie a fancy bow around her and you could've started an auction frenzy.

Not only was I feeling good, but I was eating like a horse; probably the only horse quality I would ever be compared to! I was nearing 130lbs and looking a lot better for it. I was actually beginning to feel comfortable with my body again and didn't feel too out of place standing beside my wonderful looking girl.

Mentally I had completely turned myself around. Teri hadn't really been witness to my troubled years, and only saw me for the witty and confident guy that I'd become once again.

I thought of my little imaginary friend once more, lying in his hospital bed with his shiny bald head.

Good job Brandon. I knew you could do it. It's all about wanting to win and having something to fight for. Looks like you've beat it; the future is looking bright now. I think this should be the last time we talk. You don't need me anymore.

Moving In

Teri and I had been together for almost nine months now and it was wonderful. We spent at least three nights of the week together and almost the entire weekends. There was warmth to our relationship that no doubt many couples wished they had. That was unfortunate for them, but for me everything was perfect.

My Remicade treatment was going well and I was still feeling great both mentally and physically. I was exercising every other day; nothing too strenuous, but basically a bit of walking, stretching and strengthening, and a few laps around the swimming pool. It was incredible, and a day I once thought I would never see again.

My new lease on life also had a positive affect on the cleanliness of my apartment, which was previously a festering haven for dust accumulation, molding Chinese take-out, and countless microscopic bugs that buzzed around and nibbled on my skin every chance they got. Not any more. It was clean, dust free and I'd even spread around a few of those plug in scented air fresheners in every room. I was now able to maintain the place the way it deserved, but I really made the extra effort as I didn't want Teri to see I was a complete slob. She could find that out for herself in due time!

It was a Saturday morning as we lazed around on my blue suede sofa, watching a show on the Animal Planet channel about the mating rituals of snakes. It was fascinating stuff as we munched on some reheated leftover pizza from the night before.

"How much are you paying each month on rent for your place?" I inquired.

"Too much; it's twelve hundred per month, so four hundred between the three of us. Including bills it comes out about five hundred."

"Seems like a bit of a waste considering you're never there."

"Well we can take turns on the weekends on where we stay."

"No it's OK, I don't want to have to think about keeping the noise down during the throws of passion. In saying that though, your flat mates might get off on that."

"You always have to find something crude to comment on, don't you?"

"Yeah, you know me too well. Seriously though, it does seem like a bit of a waste of money."

"So what are you suggesting?"

"Well, I've been thinking a lot about this recently. Seeing as you basically live here already, I thought that maybe you could just move in with me; if you wanted to. No pressure of course."

My heart was racing.

Please say yes, please say yes, please say yes.

There was a significant pause as she looked deep into my eyes. I couldn't figure out if she was just contemplating the idea or trying to get a read on me to determine whether I was being serious or not. It was a painful wait, so I just eyeballed her and shrugged my eyebrows and shoulders.

"I'd love to move in with you," she said excitedly, throwing her arms around me and planting a kiss on my lips, which was an interesting taste for her as I'd just slipped a piece of cheese and pepperoni into my mouth.

"You had me a little worried there," I replied, my heartbeat settling back down to a normal pace.

"I don't know why Brandon. You should know by now that I want to spend the rest of my life with you."

Golfer Again

I stood on the eighteenth tee four under par, attempting to control my mental excitement and feeling of disbelief at what was unfolding; but it was a losing battle, as the hair on my arms was standing on end. I tried to block it out and save the celebration for the nineteenth hole, but it was no good, as I sent my final tee shot into the trees on the left side of the fairway. Many years ago such a shot would've resulted in a barrage of profanities that could've turned the air blue, but not today; I was just happy to have the ability to play again.

I wearily drove the golf cart anxiously towards my tee shot. God bless South Florida for supplying carts. I was still tired, but at least able to participate. Back home golf buggies were reserved for the rich and famous or prestigious courses I was never entitled to play, but here they were as common as the number of folks walking the links back in Scotland. There was no way I'd have been able to drag my depleted joints around the five miles required for a round of golf. It was almost like fate that this day was taking place.

To my delight I had a free swing at my ball without any branches interfering, however, ahead of me was a roadblock of thick trees that could've resulted in a pinball effect should my ball come into contact with them.

The smart play was out sideways to the fairway and shoot for the green with the third shot, but where was the fun in that? Instead I set up for a final moment of glory, aiming thirty yards right of the green, taking the trees out of play, while severely hooding the face of my trusty seven iron to impart some serious right to left spin on the ball and get it bending back towards the target. It was a difficult proposition, but a much easier shot than many amateurs made it out to be. The concept was an easy one; aim the clubface where you want the ball to finish, and point your shoulders where you want the ball flight to start; then swing the club as normal along your body alignment and trust the clubface to do its job. The trust part was problem for most, as they would attempt to steer the ball like it was attached to a remote control or something, then scratch their heads in confusion when it didn't work out!

The contact I made was pure, and I watched the little white sphere sail perfectly along the first third of its journey. It was a thing of beauty as it began turning towards the planned destination.

"Keep turning baby!" I said in a fake American accent.

It was almost listening to me as it continued to curve, and landed softly on the green, no more than twenty feet from the flag; the hairs on my arms more erect than when I was on the tee box.

"Super shot chief," exclaimed Dec, as surprised as I was at actually pulling it off.

The birdie putt was a slight anti-climax as it was always wide of the hole, but stopped around six inches from the cup. I tapped in for par and a four under round of sixty-eight, and we made our way merrily to the nineteenth for a well-deserved cold beer.

I stopped at the clubhouse restroom before heading through to the lounge for some lunch and a beverage. I was in disbelief as I locked myself in one of the bathroom stalls, checking there was nobody else in the room first. I sat, head in hands and openly sobbed. This day had been a dream for a long time and even a year ago I believed it would always remain just that—a fantasy I could reflect on when looking for positive memories. Not today though; I had done it, I was back, and unlike my tears from before, these were tears of joy.

I was careful not to get too far ahead of myself though, as I knew that my current jubilation could possibly turn into disappointment with a sudden inflammation flare-up, but I knew I wanted to continue my involvement with golf, even if it wasn't on a playing level. I had a great eye for the game and mechanics of the swing, so decided to enroll in a week long intensive course to try and achieve my certified professional teacher qualification.

The association was the PGTCA (Professional Golf Teachers and Coaches of America), a highly touted organization in the monthly publication, Golf Magazine.

There were a dozen of us enrolled for the class. We anxiously sat around the large wooden oval table in the hotel conference room for our introduction meeting and course agenda.

The location was a plain, but nice-looking hotel and golf resort in Fort Myers, on the west coast of Florida. It was convenient for me as it was only about a ninety minute drive from my home, unlike many of the other participants who had driven ten hours from Georgia, or a couple of guys who had flown in from the New York area.

For me it was an expensive class to take, running at just under two thousand dollars for the week, including accommodation, but more so for those adding in flight costs.

"Welcome gentlemen. I'm Ken Williams, and will be your master instructor for the week. I'm very glad you could join us for our class A instructor certification session this week at the lovely Admiral LeHigh Resort in Fort Myers. Let me start by stating up front that this week is going to be intense, and will challenge you all mentally as well as physically. Days will be long, beginning at 7:00 am each morning and running until 3:00 pm. This time will be focused on swing mechanics, fault finding, educational drills, as well as giving instructions on how to present yourselves when giving an actual golf lesson to a paying member of the public. After 3:00 pm you will have courtesy of the resort course to play and practice as little or as much as you'd like. Let it be noted that familiarity with the golf course will be in your best interest. Friday afternoon is the playability test. It is eighteen holes of golf around the course here, and your score will be put forward towards your overall grade. Friday *morning* there is a three hour written examination. After your round of golf in the afternoon you will be required to give a practical golf lesson. I will give you a total of five situations that an amateur player may require help with. It will be up to you to deliver and show me how you would communicate and illustrate this during a real-life situation. Again, your performance in all these areas will make up your overall grade. The pass mark is 75%. It *will* be tough, and our pass rate of individuals who attend is approximately seven from ten, so a few of you will probably not achieve certification. We have to be stringent with our requirements in order to maintain the integrity of our organization. We want to have the best people out there representing the association. But rest assured, I will give you my all. I have over twenty years experience of teaching, and have delivered this class more times than I can remember. All I ask from you in return is that you give me your all. Take as many notes during the class as you need. The written test is extremely tough, so your evenings may require a few hours of study preparation. Do whatever it takes for you to get the most out of the money you are spending. That's all from me guys. I'd like to go around the table one by one, introduce yourself, where you are from, any golfing achievements, as well as your expectations from this class and what you would like to do with it should you achieve certification status."

Ken looked like he was in his early fifties. He stood about six feet tall, short grey hair and a neatly trimmed matching moustache, with his tanned skin causing the silver shininess of his hair to standout like a polar bear in the snow wearing a luminous green sweatshirt. He was dressed immaculately; Gary Player style, all in black and finely pressed. There was a confidence from him that oozed knowledge, and it was difficult to defend the idea that a lot wouldn't be learned this week.

I was used to public speaking; it was part and parcel of my job role. I'd carried out countless presentations in front of a lot more people than the amount in this room, so I delivered my introduction with ease.

"Hi guys, I'm Brandon Wilkinson, originally from the home of golf. That's Scotland for those of you trying to get past my thick American accent!"

That received some heavy laughter. My accent would've been at home on the set of Braveheart, and even recognizable to a tribe of Amazon pygmies unaccustomed to civilization

"I'm just now getting back into the game of golf after a long lay-off due to injury. I was county champion back in Scotland when I was eighteen, where I held a scratch handicap. My expectation from this class is to enhance my knowledge of the golf swing and pick up some key improvement drills for some of the most common faults amateur players suffer from. If—fingers crossed—I successfully pass the course, I'd like to land myself a part-time job giving lessons at a local course or driving range."

The introductions continued around the table in a clockwise rotation. My main concern before my arrival was that I might be out of my depth here, but that notion was swiftly squashed. I'd started a trend as far as mentioning golf handicap, and by the time Jerome—the last guy in the circle—had given his little speech, it was clear I was probably the best player; on paper anyway. I wasn't quite the player I had been before, as my stamina and mobility was now hindered, but the use of golf carts to restrict the need for walking put me right back up there.

We all made our way back to our hotel rooms. They were located outside the main building, and were terraced style rooms where the entrance doors opened directly onto the parking lot. The facility was touted as luxurious, but unless a homeless guy was writing the review, it was more than a little generous. It was clean and tidy, but no more pristine than a Motel 6 or Days Inn. There wasn't even a coffee maker, and the twenty inch screen sitting on top of the wooden dresser wasn't exactly high-tech. Still, it was neat, dry, and would serve its purpose for the week.

I'd just finished up a call to the lovely Teri when there was a heavy knock at the door, which took me a little by surprise. Not only was I not expecting anyone, but I was sitting there in only a pair of boxer shorts and a smile! I timidly opened the door about six inches and peeked out with one eye.

"Hey Brandon, we're living next door for the week and wanted to see if you were interested in a few drinks. We've got a bunch of beers on ice and were planning some cards before this class kicks off in the morning."

It was Greg and Jerome. They were part of the course and I had them tagged as the two standout characters from our induction session.

"Sounds good guys; give me ten minutes to get ready and I'll be right over. Thanks again for the invite."

Surprisingly enough I was in the mood for a beer! They were the two guys who'd made the drive down from Georgia, and had that southern style drawl to their accent that I found very entertaining; probably equivalent to the way Americans found mine fascinating.

I slipped on a pair of blue jeans and a red golf polo shirt. It was nice of them to invite me in for a drink. I wasn't sure whether it was because I was on my own or whether they heard the accent from earlier and figured "he no doubt likes a beverage." Although that would've been stereotyping my nationality, it was true in my case, and to be honest I was happy for the social interaction and the free cold beer that was going to accompany it.

"Hey Greg; how you doing?"

"Hey buddy, glad you could join us. Come on in."

The rooms were clean and tidy upon entering for the first time, but Greg and Jerome being a typical pair of guys on their own for the week had quickly removed the tidy tag in a hurry. Their suitcases were lying flipped open on the floor at the foot of each queen bed, the bathroom sink had now become the bar area, filled with ice and crammed to the top with Coors Light cans. The boys were now dressed in sweat pants and scabby looking t-shirts that were no strangers to a wear while painting or doing other odd jobs around their homes. Jerome's shirt had a Budweiser logo on it, and in true redneck fashion, Greg was sporting the words "GIT-R-DONE" on the front of his. Their smart golfing attire from the meeting earlier had been cast aside like old rags on the floor beside the open suitcases—inside-out of course.

There were an array of golf balls scattered over the floor, most of which were gathered on the dark blue carpet beside a pair of dirty white Nike sneakers that formed an open v-shape, heels together and toes pointing out at forty five degrees close to the back wall; no doubt the result of an earlier putting contest.

The beers flowed well, but the luck with the poker cards not so good. They cleaned me for twenty-five dollars, but factoring in the number of free beers consumed, I probably broke even.

I turned in around eleven thirty and must've fallen asleep within a few minutes after my head hit the pillow. I'd attempted to watch The Late Show with Jay Leno, but I awoke to the morning sunshine streaming through the vertical slit in the thick curtains and the sound of the early morning news on channel six.

I'd slept like a log, but was slightly disappointed I'd missed Jay's interview with Sandra Bullock. There was just something about her that got my juices flowing. She wasn't completely gorgeous, but her witty and bubbly personality elevated her—in my opinion—way beyond your Cindy Crawford and Naomi Campbell super model types.

The first day of class was finally over, and as initially presented to us, it was extremely intense. My hand was as stiff as a claw as a result of the number of lines I'd scribbled in my notebook. I chuckled to myself after Ken told us we were done for the day. I felt as though I'd beaten arthritis, but if the next four days continued like this, I'd probably have another dose in my right hand from the frantic note taking.

After class, Greg, Jerome and I headed to the first tee for some practice. I was mentally exhausted, but knew I had to familiarize myself with the course as it was forming part of the examination.

It was closing in on four thirty, but the sun was still blazing. I was on my second shirt, but even that was so drenched in sweat it looked as though it had been applied to my body with dark red paint.

We putted out on the ninth hole and called it a day, deciding to head back to the nineteenth hole—their beer filled sink as opposed to the clubhouse.

The plan was to study later in the evening, but my mind was completely wiped out from the intensity of the day. Four beers in the boys place and I retired to my room for a nap; after calling Teri and giving her the rundown of the first day.

I awoke, reasonably refreshed, but still not in the mood for any studying. The day had more or less covered the fundamentals anyway, which I was already knowledgeable of, so I decided a relaxing wind down at the hotel bar was the order of the evening.

I made the short walk to the bar area. My joints ached a little, but I'd been on my feet for much of the day, so I was probably in line with most of the other guys in the group.

To my surprise, Ken Williams and his assistant Sergio were sitting bar side as I walked in. Ken even looked immaculate with a Bud Light in his hand and a Marlboro hanging out of his mouth.

"Evening gents," I said, taking the stool directly beside them.

"Mr. Wilkinson, how are you? Nice performance today."

I could tell what he was referring to, and although I thought I'd executed well, it was great to hear it from the horse's mouth.

Ken had been describing how to execute certain shots; hitting them high, low, hooking and slicing, and had asked me to follow his instructions and attempt to demonstrate the shots on the driving range. I was sure he'd selected me as I was the best player on paper. I was a little nervous in front of the group, but it was a situation in tournament play I'd dealt with many years before, and I'd played these shots so often in the past, especially in Scotland where shaping the ball in the howling wind was essentially a prerequisite to success.

I nailed every one of them, and instantly gained the respect of my peers, some of whom were no doubt eager to see if my scratch handicap was genuine or an attempt to gain attention.

"Thanks Ken, I really appreciate that."

"Seriously though, that was some impressive ball striking."

"I surprised myself a little. I've hit all of them a thousand times, but I've only been seriously practicing again for the last few months."

We drank the night away, exchanging a variety of old golf stories. The bar was quiet when I arrived, but it had filled up rather quickly with what appeared to be some of the locals from the surrounding area. They all knew one another and were on first name terms with the bar staff.

The local patrons appeared to be stuck in a time warp; all dressed in long sleeved shirts with collars on them fit for a giant's wardrobe, and bell bottom pants so tight around the crotch you could almost see a detailed imprint of their meat and two veg.

As it turned out it was seventies Karaoke night. Ken, Sergio, and myself had been ready to leave, but decided another round of drinks was in order so we could get a glimpse of a few of the performers.

The décor of the bar matched the Karaoke theme. The brown and beige retro style wallpaper reminded me of my grandmother's living room when I was a small boy. The lights were now dimmed and I was almost blinded periodically as the spinning disco lights reflected from the globe-sized glitter ball hanging on the ceiling directly above the snooker table sized dance floor.

"Ladies and gentlemen, opening for us this evening is Jerry with his take on the Beatles classic Help," came the magnified words from the dorky looking MC for the evening, who obviously was attempting to make up for a previously non-accomplished ambition of being a radio DJ.

The song Jerry picked to give a rendition on was well chosen, as he certainly sounded like he needed help. He must've been out elsewhere for a few beverages before he made it to the hotel bar, as he slurred his way through the song and struggled to keep up with the timing of the words on the autocue, much to the amusement of his friends, and even more so for Ken, Sergio, and myself.

We finished up our drinks and reluctantly left the bar, as it was just beginning to get interesting, but there was much work to be done this week and I had to remain fairly focused.

The next three days were equally intense; not only on the mind, but on the body as well, and a real test for me. This was as much of an examination for me as tomorrow's testing, and I was mentally boosted by the fact that my joints appeared to be in as good a shape as they had been at the beginning of the week.

It was Thursday evening and tomorrow was the big day. For the first time in the week I decided that some *intense* studying combined with a good night's sleep was the way to go instead of propping up the bar.

"OK gentlemen, you have three hours to complete the following paper," announced Ken calmly; no doubt a lot calmer than the rest of us about to endure the long winded test.

Surprisingly I found it a breeze. There were a few tricky questions, but the previous night's learning had turned out to be an extremely smart decision.

The day was far from over though. Next up was the playability test, and we all made our way wearily to the first tee. My brain was still throbbing. It has been fairly easy, but it had been a long drawn out affair and did require a lot of thought. I wasn't particularly enthused about going straight into between four or five hours in the baking sun, but there was no choice in the matter. Fortunately there was a breeze picking up, and although it was still smoking hot, it did offer a small amount of reprieve.

Like a professional golfing event, we were announced individually onto the first tee. We were playing in four separate groups of three, and a small mixed crowd of folks from the local club and others on vacation had congregated to watch this bunch of potential golf teachers stripe a drive up the middle of the tight fairway.

The onlookers appeared a little perplexed. The strokes from the opening two groups were more than a million miles away from a Tiger Woods stinger traveling speedily along what appeared to be an invisible length of rope.

You could almost cut the tension in the air with a knife, and this was ultimately impacting the quality of the golf seen so far. This was a big moment for us all, especially as the overall pass or fail for this arduous week could rest on this particular performance.

"On the tee, Brandon Wilkinson," uttered the polite tone from Ken Williams, followed by some polite applause from the members of the audience that still remained, even after the disappointment from the first two groups.

This was my time to shine.

Come on kid, you can do this.

I took a few deep breaths, mainly to compose myself, but also to give enough time for the hairs on my arms to return to a flaccid state, as they had been standing on end with excitement.

It had been many years since I'd experienced an adrenalin rush like this, but I dug deep into past success in such situations and regained my focus.

The ball left my clubface like a bullet, and missed the center of the short grass by a matter of inches. There was louder applause, and I sent an appreciative tip of my baseball cap in the general direction of the onlookers.

I was surprisingly calm, but I'd decided to take a "couldn't care less" attitude for the day.

Relax, have fun, and whatever happens is meant to be. Holy crap, you never thought this day would've ever taken place, so think yourself lucky to even be here.

Ken had set the groupings for the day and had conveniently paired me with Greg and Jerome, which was a relaxing component by itself. Greg took everything in his stride and was an excellent ball striker. Jerome was not as naturally gifted, but what he lacked in ability he made up with character and sheer determination. It was going to be a fun day.

It all went as planned, and the three of us fully settled down after around three holes and treated it as a normal weekend game of fun with the boys. We fed off each other and cruised around, our scores well under the course requirement, and I took the "gold medal" as they called it, although there wasn't *actually* a trophy for the best score.

We jadedly filtered back to the driving range to complete the final element of the week—the practical lesson presentation. It was hard to maintain motivation.

It had been almost five hours to complete the eighteen holes. The two groups in front of us had been snail like in pace, lining up putts from every perceivable angle and taking an eternity for club selection between shots. It was an important day, but you would've thought they were participating in the final pairings of the U.S. Open—with the exception of the disappointing scores they turned in. However, we could now see the end of the week on the horizon, so it was time to dig deep and see it out until conclusion. There would be plenty of time to rest afterwards.

The lesson presentation went equally well. I could tell from Ken's facial expressions that I'd carried out a good job.

The week was finally over and we sat attentively as Ken read out the results.

"I'm going to read out the top three performers. The remainder of you can see me personally for your grade."

This signaled to me that not everyone had been successful, and he wasn't going to publicly humiliate those on the wrong side of the fence, which was a classy touch in my opinion.

"Taking top place with a total score of 94% is Brandon Wilkinson."

My heart pounded as I made my way to Ken for the customary handshake, and posed for a quick photograph taken by Sergio. It had the feeling of a miniature graduation ceremony, and I literally had to fight back the joyful tears.

It was all over and I packed my case after saying goodbye to my eleven friends from the week.

As I changed into some fresh clothes and bundled my sweat stained ones from the day into a plastic shopping bag, my emotions got the better of me. I was alone in my room and could finally let it all out, even although I still tried to fight the urge.

Come on son, get a grip on yourself.

It was no use, especially as my little friend popped back into my mind.

Let it out Brandon. You deserve the release. Your efforts to beat your illness finally have something tangible to attach to. Enjoy the moment.

I'd thought our previous encounter might be the final one, but I needed the ultimate confirmation from my little leukemia stricken buddy to make it all seem appropriate. I was going to miss his little bald optimistic head.

I completely lost it, falling face first onto the bed, sobbing like a wounded child, attempting to muffle my wailing with the freshly cleaned floral patterned quilt. They were happy tears, but tears nevertheless. I *really* never believed I'd have swung a golf club again, never mind taking top honors at a professional teacher's course. The realization of basically being a normal human being again was hitting home like a power drill on an asphalt road. It was completely overwhelming, but I was a lucky, lucky man, and the future was definitely bright.

Finally on Track

It was like a dream come true. Life was good again; different, but good nevertheless. I'd fought through the depression and pain, and was now holding the ultimate prize. So what if I couldn't do a spinning roundhouse kick like I used to. The only time that was ever used was when Jean-Claude Van Damme slowly and deliberately delivered one to the side of a thug's head while his hooligan friends waited patiently in line to receive their own individual ass beating, rather than all of them rushing the "Muscles from Brussels" and kicking his ass; hardly real life and never exactly practical.

In addition, I was fine with not being able to sprint one hundred meters in less than fifteen seconds, or sprint at all for that matter. Other than competing in high school track and field or running to catch a bus, this was another capability that was rarely called upon. School was long gone and I owned my own transportation, so why should I be concerned.

The fact I had now accepted my limitations was life changing. I was pain free, but still constrained with what I could do. My life had been adapted now and I was comfortable with my new routine.

I now weighed in at an impressive 155lbs, which for my five foot six stature was respectable in anyone's book. It was a long way removed from my gaunt skeleton looking frame where I would've been at home as a tribe member of an Ethiopian village.

I reflected often, almost like an out of body experience at times. When my mind reproduced my painful and troubling times, it was like I was hovering in grandeur above the previous crippled image of myself, watching in pity as this sorry soul dragged himself wearily along a journey of hell. It was as though I'd migrated through an overly successful reincarnation process.

I was now mentally strong; easily as equivalent to the physical traits of a professional street fighter. Like this counterpart, I had my physical scars, but also my inner scars. It had been a long journey of lessons learned, and I was as ready as ever to take on the world.

There was a knock on affect throughout my life. Not only did I believe I looked healthier, but I felt that way inside as well, had a fantastic woman by my side, and received a promotion at work; all aspects that boosted my state of mind and no doubt contributed to the remission of my disease, even if I could never scientifically prove that.

The new drug obviously fitted *heavily* into the mathematical improvement model, but in my mind there was a combination of factors that optimized the response variable, and I had the settings dialed in at maximum output.

Being an optimistic and bubbly character again suited me, and spilled over to my rejuvenated exercise regime; swimming every other day and working on low intensity weight machines. I was again the life and soul of the party at social events and I just loved being alive again.

It was a transition that everybody close to me never thought would come.

Present Day

Night and day, black and white, chalk and cheese; pick one, they all represent the magnitude of transformation.

Those meeting me now for the first time had no idea, and probably never would, unless they became close enough to me and I felt the urge to fill them in on my troubled past.

I had been having a cup of coffee one day with a colleague from the office in the work cafeteria. A group of guys I'd seen around before but didn't know too well were walking past and must've heard my Scottish accent.

"Excuse me. Sorry to interrupt, but are you from Scotland?"

"Yes, I am," I replied, a little baffled by the introduction.

"Hi I'm Duane; I work in the Development Engineering team. I've seen you walking around the factory a few times recently, but I had no idea you were Scottish. I am the captain of the company's soccer team. We need one more person to fill this season's roster and I know that the game is really big from where you are from. So I was wondering if you played, and if so, whether you would like to join the team?"

"Hi Duane, I'm Brandon. I would love to, but I had hip surgery a while back and I'm still having a few knee problems. I love the game and normally would gladly say yes, but my body right now just couldn't handle the punishment. I do appreciate the offer though."

"No problem Brandon. Listen, if you change your mind, just let me know next time you see me around."

"I will do. Thanks again."

Obviously I had to decline, but that moment will stick in my head forever. To Duane I must've looked fit and healthy enough to participate, and it was a stark realization that I did appear in good shape to others and it wasn't just a hopeful façade spinning around in a delusional mind.

As I write this final chapter, I reflect back on the multitude of emotions that have been a rollercoaster ride I'll never forget. I'm now thirty three, and it's rather fitting that it's been just over a decade to the day since the events of the first chapter.

My previous paranoia, self-consciousness, and days of extreme depression and pain have turned full circle into that of self-confidence, pride, and satisfaction. I have a very fulfilling and fantastic family life, as well as a highly successful corporate career that has provided an awesome salary and many lifestyle luxuries that I could never have fathomed ten years ago.

The irony of it all is that I'm convinced I wouldn't be the success I am today without all the mental, emotional and physical pain. To say it has molded me into the strong and triumphant man I have become would be the understatement of the century.

As I type at this very moment, I am gazing out—pain free—over the swimming pool in the backyard of my Florida home. It's a warm day and the sun is shining; in the sky above and also in my heart. My two dogs are running around without a care in the world, playing tug of war with a pair of my—used to be favorite—boxer shorts. Not leaving laundry around needs to be added to the "to-do" list. The Great Dane looks as happy as a pig in shit, even though she herself seems to be developing arthritis in the right hip of her hind leg. Is she going to lie down and give in to it all? Of course not, and neither should anyone out there, young or old. Life is a journey, often a painful one in so many ways, with obstacles thrown in our way at the most inconvenient of times, strategically placed to challenge our character. Never give up—*ever*!

Mental strength is everything, and can often be the most effective drug in relieving pain and emotional turmoil. Never isolate those who love you—they love you for a reason. In the case of arthritis, remain as active as possible, push *hard* for the latest advancements in medical care, but most of all, keep a positive mental attitude—a cure may just be around the corner. In times of strife, visualize my imaginary leukemia stricken teenage friend, counting down the days until his journey to heaven, or picture some of the starving kids in Africa with their swollen malnourished stomachs and flies buzzing around their desperate faces. Things can always be worse, and these types of images really does put everything into perspective, so be thankful for friends and family. Take every step you can to beat this disease—it *can* be done.

Find a combination of tasks and actions that work for *you*. Everyone is different, so persevere. It may take a considerable amount of time to find the right one, and trial and error is very likely the only route. Create a daily journal; note what activities you completed, food you ate, medications taken, as well as detailing your general mood throughout the day and any significant occurrences that lead to that state of mind.

From my journal entries I've created the following list of issues encountered, things worth trying, as well as a few mental aspects and *possible* solutions. Many of these experiences and traits could be common to all chronic pain sufferers.

1. Closeness Issues

    This is an area that *may* be unique to a small percentage of sufferers, but I was in that bucket until fairly recently. Closeness issues affect all types of people, even the perfectly healthy. The fear of rejection for some can create issues of this nature. I found it was easier to keep people at a distance, particularly when there was potential for any physical contact. Like several of the relationships described in the previous pages, it was the fear of not only being hurt again, but being hurt or cast aside as a result of my condition. The fear of being a burden to somebody should I deteriorate and require assistance even for the simplest tasks such as taking a leak was a real one, and easier just to avoid altogether.

    I still fight this to a degree today, but I am much better now that I have my wife by my side. She has been so wonderful and never considered the arthritis anything more than an unfortunate situation that we just had to work through.

    On that note, just take a chance; those who love and care for you will always be around. Those who jump ship weren't worth having around in the first place. Better to discover sooner than later, so don't hold back.

2. Push the Doctor

    Don't take that literally! Seriously though, just do it and don't be shy. It's like the old phrase; you don't ask you don't get.

    My encounters with rheumatologists have been nothing but positive, and I cannot say enough good things about Dr. Kapila who I am still seeing to this day. They are all generally nice, caring people who *want* to help you. It's their job, but their actions can only be as effective as the feedback you provide them during periodic check-ups.

    Please don't make the mistake I did, before finally giving myself a good kick up the ass. I was never the type to complain. At times if a drug wasn't helping I just assumed that that was the way it was going to be. It doesn't have to be; there are many alternative options out there that can be explored. During appointments years ago I was always asked how I'd been feeling since the last time. My usual response was "not too bad." This type of feedback is normally interpreted as an indicator that things are not deteriorating, so the decision is usually to continue on "as is." My opinion now is that "not bad" means "not good" or "could be better." Swallow your pride and be open; they are there to hear your problems. If a drug isn't leading to improvement then let them know. Ask to try something new, quiz them on whether there are any new treatments available that are showing good results in clinical trials. Push the envelope until you find what works for you. As I said, they want to assist, but you need to be honest and open in order to initiate change.

3. Positive Mental Attitude

I cannot stress the importance of this enough. It might be the most difficult to maintain at times, and there *will* be ups and downs, but as long as the peaks outweigh the troughs, you're on the right track.

I found that my pain levels were heavily influenced by mood. They say laughter is the best medicine. Obviously it wouldn't be as good as a drug that cured the disease, but there is a lot to be said for it. I started to watch a lot of TV sit-coms and even frequented the local comedy club on a regular basis. This improved my demeanor ten fold, and combined with knowing I was still more fortunate than many with terminal conditions, as well as the homeless and starving, rammed home the point that things weren't all that bad and I was still surrounded by loving friends and family for support. Sure, things could always be better, but we can say that about all facets of life, from what we do for a living, to general financial status.

4. Experiment with Diet

This is not something that made a huge difference for me, but it's definitely worth mentioning. I've read so many success stories in this area that it cannot be discounted.

I now essentially just eat healthier. Previously I could hardly bring myself to drive past a McDonalds. Maximize the fresh fruit and vegetables and eliminate as much of the processed products high in artificial additives. The main benefit I found was an increased energy level. Previously I became lethargic very easily, and this could alter my mood; but not any longer.

I've read several articles where people with arthritic pain have completely revamped their eating habits and are now living pain free. By all means give it a try; it *could* be the missing piece of the puzzle that completes *your* personal jigsaw. If you don't try all possibilities, you'll never know if it would've worked or not.

5.   Exercise

My thoughts in this chapter can be transposed to many medical conditions, but exercise is a crucial element to combat arthritis. I'm not for one minute suggesting you become a daily feature at the local gym, but develop a routine that you are comfortable with. Age and advancement of your disease are (in my mind) the main restrictors. Find what works for you, but keep moving, lubricate those joints. Doing nothing will never improve stiffness. It's like anything in life; if nothing is changed, why would there ever be a different end result?

For me, daily stretching combined with 10-15 minutes of low impact exercise is enough. By low impact I mean activities that put little or no stress on the joints. I find swimming to be the best, but these elliptical machines are good, and I also invested in a product known as a Total Gym that was advertised on TV by Chuck Norris, which has been absolutely fantastic in aiding my progression. It'll never turn me into Chuck, but it has certainly contributed to the new me.

6.   Massage

This is a fairly recent addition for me, but one that certainly provided benefit in terms of muscle relaxation as opposed to joint mobility.

My muscles continue to develop and are not completely where I want them to be. As a result of this they become more easily fatigued compared to normal healthy men of my age. It's not a major issue in the grand scheme of things, but the occasional ache is something I like to avoid if possible.

Massage has been a fantastic outlet to relieve this irritation. My wife suggested we take up membership at a new health spa that had opened in our local area. I wasn't so sure about paying a monthly fee for something I may not use, but agreed to go as there was a free trial offer that was being dangled like bait in the newspaper ads section, and my wife was all over it like a ravenous piranha.

After our first session I finally admitted to my wife that it had been an excellent idea and she gave me the "I told you so" response. Of course, my decision making hadn't been influenced by the array of gorgeous female staff, or specifically Liliana, the stunning Latin girl who'd been rubbing me all over with hot oils for an hour!

Kidding aside, this is worth exploring. I find it one of the best relaxation techniques around. It frees my mind as I lie there, soft sounds of the ocean playing in the background, and comforted by the thought that any knots in my back or shoulders created by my slightly skewed posture, will soon be gone.

7. <u>Stand Up and Fight</u>

This is *so* closely linked to positive mental attitude; in fact they are not disjointed. Standing up and fighting is the only way to boost your mind set. There will always be fears, but meet them head on. A particular condition may never be eradicated, but think of steps that can be taken to adjust.

I'll never be the athlete I once was, but I have substituted the martial arts and soccer with swimming, golf, pool and darts. I can do these well, and quite the man to beat at the local bar when it comes to the latter two.

If you had a fear of heights, I'd suggest a trip to the top of the Empire State building or Eiffel Tower. Meet your fears head on and take whatever steps necessary to eliminate. Being a quitter will only lead to deterioration.

8. <u>Socialize</u>

This is *extremely* relevant to fighting your disease as well as your fears. The head on approach *is* the way to go.

From what you have read in previous chapters, this was a big issue for me, as I would lock myself away at times like a prisoner in solitary confinement. I didn't want people's pity or even strangers looking at my struggles. This only resulted in depression and negative thoughts. Grab the bull by the horns. Screw what people think; you are who you are.

I joined my local pool team as an avenue to "get back out there." Sure, most folks asked me what was wrong with my legs, but be upfront and tell them. You will get looks that tell you they feel sorry for you, or even verbal replies like "I'm sorry to hear that." Face that head on as well and let them know you are fine with it. Say it with a smile; that's what I did. It genuinely impresses people that you show such courage. I've even had people saying they wished they could be more like *me*, as far as being able to deal with adversity in their lives.

After a while in a particular social environment, people stop noticing your condition. A friend of mine used to have long, crazy-looking hair and an equally as wild beard. One day he showed up at the bar clean shaven with a number one buzz cut. He took so many jibes about it all, but within a week or so it never even entered any discussions. The point is that familiarity quickly becomes the norm.

However, I did start receiving some further comments, all positives though. As I progressed with my exercise regime, improved diet, a good attitude and the right medication combination, I not only looked and felt better, but actually appeared more mobile. This was noticed by all my acquaintances and only encouraged me even more to succeed.

Ask any woman who has been fighting to control their weight. If they lose 20-30 lbs via exercise and diet, and begin to receive compliments on how good they look, they'll tell you how great it makes them feel and that it's probably the single best motivation factor in order to make the lifestyle changes an integral part of their routine going forward.

9.   Ask for Help if You Need It

Hopefully many of you out there are not as stubborn and pig-headed as I used to be. There are times to do things yourself of course, but certain cir-cumstances require biting the bullet and asking for help.

I learned my lesson the hard way as I tried to pretend I was normal and could do even the most strenuous of tasks on my own—what a complete fool. Lift-ing furniture for even the fittest of folks can be rather demanding, but a frail, joint damaged young man with thigh muscles that had been posted missing in action was basically a formula for disaster.

My knees were messed up for over a month—ligament damage. I had a mul-titude of friends who would've helped me, and they were extremely pissed off when they found out how idiotic I'd been.

It's not that you *can't* perform difficult tasks; it just doesn't make sense to do so. I lifted the table and chair set as well as the TV, but I paid for it afterwards. Swallow your pride and ask for help. It doesn't make you any less of a person.

10. <u>The Winning Combination</u>

This entire concept is like a guy with the kitchen skills of Homer Simpson being handed a bunch of cooking ingredients, no instructions, and being asked to make a cake that tastes fantastic. The first attempt will likely be a complete disaster, but after messing around over time with a few combinations, chances are you'll be able to create something that is extremely edible.

The same is true with arthritis. Keep adding ingredients to try, remove others that seem ineffective, work on combinations. It might take a while to make that prize-winning cake, but persist; Rome wasn't built in a day.

The above ten points should be given consideration. One of them may be the answer or some blend of them all. Keep close track of what works and build upon it.

For those reading these words that are experiencing hell right now please stay strong; work at it and fight until the end. It *can* be done and I'm living proof.

There's a minute left in the game, and the clock is ticking on this closely fought scoreless match. The anxiety in the crowd makes it feel like an opposition player is chasing me down. I see the faces of my parents magnify from the thousands in attendance like a bad hallucination, their grief stricken frowns signaling to me that they're terrified, unsure which direction my life is going to take; their slow-trickling tears being the only encouragement I need.

Arthritis has the ball, and making its way like a charging rush of inflammation towards my goal line. Oh no you don't! This may be the final game of my life and I'm going down fighting. A sliding tackle that David Beckham would've been proud of courageously wins back the ball. Arthritis is down, but the referee signals play on. Arthritis looks beaten, and I can almost feel my adrenalin neutralize the inflammatory bastard. My joints are loosening with each step as I near the eighteen yard box, maintaining close ball control as I see the referee scrutinize his watch. I let loose an almighty shot—postage stamp, top corner of the net, get it up you! The sound of the final whistle is almost lost in the jubilation of the crowd, friends and family invading the field, minds now at ease with the glorious outcome. Me 1 Arthritis 0.

978-0-595-48824-7
0-595-48824-2

www.ingramcontent.com/pod-product-compliance
Lightning Source LLC
Chambersburg PA
CBHW030322290526
45785CB00001B/473